MINI SAGA IN SOUTH AFRICA

HILARY CROWLEY

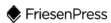

One Printers Way
Altona, MB R0G 0B0
Canada

www.friesenpress.com

Copyright © 2023 by Hilary Crowley
First Edition — 2023

1815 Adams Rd Summit Lake, British Columbia
www.hilarycrowleyauthor.ca

All rights reserved.

No part of this publication may be reproduced in any form, or by any means, electronic or mechanical, including photocopying, recording, or any information browsing, storage, or retrieval system, without permission in writing from FriesenPress.

All photos by author, unless otherwise stated.
Maps developed by Jean-Yves Landry. www.humanecology.ca

ISBN
978-1-03-918176-2 (Hardcover)
978-1-03-918175-5 (Paperback)
978-1-03-918177-9 (eBook)

1. TRAVEL, AFRICA, REPUBLIC OF SOUTH AFRICA

Distributed to the trade by The Ingram Book Company

Dedication

Dedicated to the memory of Nelson Mandela and to Father Trevor Huddleston and all the great activists, Black and White, who helped bring an end to Apartheid in South Africa.

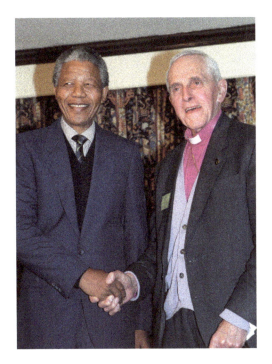

Nelson Mandela and Father Trevor Huddleston
Copyright Alamy

TABLE OF CONTENTS

ACKNOWLEDGEMENTS vii

PROLOGUE ix

1. DEPARTURE UK TO SOUTH AFRICA 1

2. PIETERMARITZBURG 11

3. ARRIVAL IN DURBAN 16

4. LESOTHO AND THE DRAKENSBERG 25

5. APARTHEID 34

6. NATAL TO THE CAPE VIA THE GARDEN ROUTE 43

7. CAPE TOWN 51

8. GROOTE SCHUUR 56

9. SOUTH WEST AFRICA 64

10. CAPE TOWN TO JOHANNESBURG VIA
    KIMBERLEY AND LESOTHO 69

11. JOHANNESBURG TO SWAZILAND 75

12. KRUGER NATIONAL PARK 80

13. BARAGWANATH 89

14. MAGALIESBERG MOUNTAINS 94

15. VOORTREKKERS 101

16. FLOCKFIELD GAME FARM 104

17. RHODESIA. 110

18. RETURN TO NATAL AND DRAKENSBERG 121

19. LEAVING SOUTH AFRICA 126

EPILOGUE 130

GLOSSARY: 135

PEOPLE FEATURED IN TEXT:. 137

GEOGRAPHICAL NAME CHANGES: 138

ABOUT THE AUTHOR 139

ACKNOWLEDGEMENTS

I have many people to thank for helping to bring this book to fruition. First must be Penny, who shared all these experiences with me. She provided the Mini, which took us around the country and provided many adventures. She also read the manuscript in its early stages to help jog my memories.

I'd like to thank my sister, Helen Roberts, for reading the manuscript in its early stages and providing her encouragement. Also my husband, Floyd, for listening to my reading, both early and late, and for providing helpful advice.

I am indebted to Dr Taru Manyanga from Zimbabwe and Dr Simon Earl from South Africa for reading and providing invaluable inputs from a Black Zimbabwean and White South African point of view. Also Dr Charles Helm, who read some early chapters and offered helpful advice.

Author Mike Nash and Nurse Judy Lett provided critical inputs on my manuscript, which I incorporated into the latest version. All these people have helped to strengthen the telling of this story, and for this, I am most grateful.

Sadly, most of the characters mentioned in this book have now passed on, but without them, there would be no story to tell, so I am indebted to them for these rich life experiences.

Thank you to Jean-Yves Landry of www.humanecology.ca who made the maps for me.

PROLOGUE

When Hilary was still in high school in England, Father Trevor Huddleston came to her girls' boarding school, St Margaret's, Bushey, and preached a sermon on South Africa. This sermon was momentous. It had a profound effect on Hilary and created a desire in her to go to Africa. He illustrated his talk with pictures and explained to the girls the injustices of forced racial segregation in South Africa. Father Huddleston told them stories of his work teaching African children in Sophiatown and about how the government brought in a Bantu Education Act disallowing African children to attend these mission schools.

He taught the students the importance of enriching these children's lives so they could strive for future success. He explained the need for ensuring the children had enough to eat so they had energy for their studies. He asked the St Margaret's students to reflect on their lives and compare them with the difficulties of African children in South Africa.

Hilary thought about this sermon for a long time. Many years later, after she had graduated from high school and became a physiotherapist, she worked at the Royal Free Hospital in London but still had a desire to go to Africa.

After work one day, when playing tennis with a physio colleague, Penny, they both expressed a wish to go to South Africa. During their game, they made impromptu plans for travel. This story covers their adventures and explorations and illustrates how life was in South Africa under Apartheid in the 1960s.

Father Trevor Huddleston, who preached that one sermon at their Church of England school in 1958, became renowned for his anti-Apartheid activism. You never know how instances in your younger life may affect your life in years to come. Hilary was raised as a non-conformist Christian but was confirmed at St Margaret's into the Anglican Church at the age of twelve. Religion was an important part of the school with scripture being one of the compulsory subjects. The students attended chapel twice a day as well as every Sunday, and Hilary had ideas of becoming a missionary, but this didn't materialise. She joined the Florence Nightingale Society and started wearing a Lady with the Lamp tiepin on her school tie, for which she was teased by her parents.

This story gives one white person's perspective on life in South Africa while Nelson Mandela was incarcerated on Robben Island.

Many name changes have taken place since Hilary was there: Rhodesia is now Zimbabwe, Salisbury is Harare, and Natal is now KwaZulu Natal. Lesotho used to be Basutoland and South West Africa is now Namibia. Hilary has mostly used the names of the places as they were when she was there in 1967–68, and she has included a glossary to capture these changes. This situates this account in its time in history and should in no way be construed as support for retention of the colonial names.

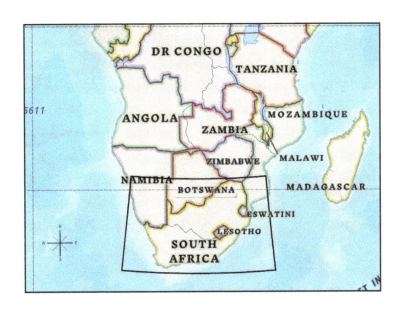

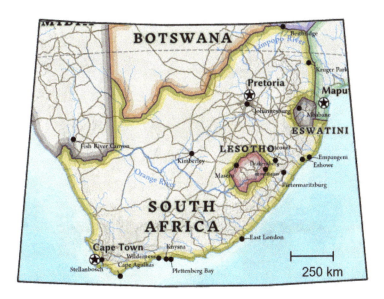

Map of South Africa, showing location

CHAPTER 1

DEPARTURE UK TO SOUTH AFRICA

*F*ather Trevor Huddleston's memorable sermon first sparked my interest in going to Africa. He impressed on me the plight of disadvantaged children raised in Apartheid South Africa compared to our privileged lives in a boarding school in England. This sermon stirred a deep interest and kindled a desire to experience Africa for myself. At some stage, shortly after leaving high school, I abandoned my thoughts of becoming a missionary, but I still had a strong desire to go to Africa.

I remembered how many years earlier, when I was still at school, I'd had a conversation with my uncle. We were gathered around my grandfather's deathbed.

Uncle Fred said to me, "What do you want to do when you leave school?"

I replied, "I haven't decided yet, but I'd like to work overseas in Africa."

He replied, "Oh, you don't want to do that. Go to America or Canada or Australia. There are lots of opportunities there, and you could make lots of money."

I said, "I'm not interested in going to those countries. My heart is set on Africa."

I made up my mind early in life that I didn't want to marry into money. I loved Uncle Fred dearly, but he was rich and drove a Rolls-Royce, and I could tell that many people in the community were envious of him. We struggled a little financially as a family, but I think it made us appreciate everything more. We never went overseas for holidays but enjoyed hiking or seaside holidays in England.

After graduating from St Margaret's School, I trained as a physiotherapist at St Thomas' Hospital in London, which was founded by Florence Nightingale. I then worked at the Royal Free Hospital in Hampstead, where I met Penny, another physiotherapist. After work one day, we were playing tennis and discussed our future plans.

I said to Penny, "What will you do after leaving the Royal Free?"

She replied, "I want to go to South Africa, where my cousin and uncle's family live."

"That's amazing!" I replied. "I also want to go to South Africa. I've yearned to go there ever since hearing Father Trevor Huddleston back at school. Where does your cousin live? Do you think we could get jobs there as physiotherapists?"

Penny replied, "My cousin, Rosemary, lives in Pietermaritzburg in Natal. Her grandfather was archdeacon of Zululand. I've always wanted to go there to visit. We could find out about work opportunities. I walk by a travel agent on my way home, so I could check on the cost of flights."

"Okay," I replied. "This is exciting. I'm sure we should be able to find physio jobs there, and we could work our way around the country. My father's sister, Eileen, lives in Cape Town, so I'm sure we could stay there too."

We continued playing tennis as we discussed these possibilities. After completing a couple of sets, we walked home to our separate abodes. Thoughts bubbled through my head as I light-footedly returned to my flat, half an hour's walk away. I couldn't wait to tell my flatmates about this enticing opportunity.

The next morning at work, as soon as I saw Penny, she said, "I provisionally booked our flights to Durban on a year's return ticket. The flight is booked for November twentieth. I didn't have to put down a deposit so thought it couldn't hurt to make the provisional reservations."

"What?" I replied. "I can't believe it. I'll have to let my parents know, but let's do it! We'll have to give in our notice at the hospital and start saving money. How exciting!"

Penny was a casual friend. She was tall and slim with dark hair. We didn't have a lot in common except we both enjoyed tennis and, as it turned out, had a desire to go to South Africa. She was friendly and unassuming, and we soon got to know each other well.

Our departure on 20 November was still two months away. Penny and I continued work at the Royal Free Hospital and started making plans for our imminent departure. We decided to travel on return tickets that were valid up to one year. Now I was going to fulfill my dream of going to Africa.

The next time I went home to Grimsby, I told my parents of our plans, and they didn't put up any serious complaints.

My mother said, "Please promise you won't marry there and will come back home after a year."

"Don't worry, Mum," I replied. "I'll come home after a year, and I have no plans to marry. I have no desire to stay in South Africa beyond the year. I love England and will stay here."

Dad said, "It's good to take advantage of every opportunity that comes your way. We'll miss you, but Auntie Eileen will be happy to see you. Make sure you write regular letters home."

I gave them a big hug and promised to write weekly letters home.

We made these provisional reservations for South Africa on 20 September 1967. We had to get yellow fever vaccinations as well as ensure all our other vaccinations were up to date. I renewed my passport, but we didn't need visas. Social life in London was always hectic, and I gradually wound down activities and bade farewell to my friends.

My father's sister, Eileen, lived in Cape Town with Auntie Daisy, who wasn't actually an aunt but a friend of Dad's mother. Her name was Daisy Solomon, daughter of the governor of the Cape. She became a suffragette in England, demanding women's right to vote, and was imprisoned for her efforts. The family also were proponents of multiracial government in South Africa so were considered radicals.

Auntie Eileen married an Afrikaner in England, Bill duPlessis. They farmed in Hertfordshire but were not successful farmers, so they had to sell the farm and move to Cornwall where they bought a confectionery store and lived above it in comparative poverty. When husband Bill died, Eileen moved in with our family and worked for my father in his wholesale tobacco and confectionary business.

After several years, she decided to emigrate to South Africa to spend time with the rest of the duPlessis family. She wound up marrying Bill's brother, Louis. This was a staunch Afrikaner family who were Calvinists and strongly supported the Nationalist Party and Apartheid. When her second husband died, Eileen moved in with Auntie Daisy and spent the rest of her days living there at St. James on the False Bay side of the Cape peninsular

Before leaving for South Africa, my mother and I took the train up to London and met Penny and her mother there for coffee. It was important for our parents to meet so they could be more confident about our imminent travels away from home. Our mothers got along well together and shared their fears and hopes. Penny's father was an architect, and the family was quite artistic. Penny's Uncle Ken was a canon in Pietermaritzburg and Zululand. My sister also had a good friend in Pietermaritzburg, Martin Prosser, so my mother was comforted by these various connections.

After hugging our parents goodbye, Penny and I flew to South Africa on a Britannia prop plane from Stansted airport, London. We flew via Basle, Tunis, and Luanda, flying over the Alps and the Sahara to Lourenco Marques in Mozambique.

We flew relatively low, so clearly saw the Alps before flying over the Mediterranean and over the Sahara Dessert. The plane even circled around Mt Kilimanjaro for us, so we got a spectacular view of the crater on top. This total flight took twenty hours, with fuel stops in Tunis and Luanda before landing in Mozambique.

On landing in Lourenco Marques, the capital of Mozambique, the feeling of arrival in Africa was immediate. As soon as we stepped out of the plane onto the tarmac, I breathed in the air, which could only be Africa's: hot, humid, and exciting. We stayed overnight there. The drive from the airport to the hotel took us through a shanty town, with makeshift houses of corrugated iron and tarpaulins, before emerging onto the city streets lined with flowering purple jacaranda and scarlet flame trees. We then drove through typical Portuguese architecture, Portugal being the colonising country of Mozambique. I was shocked at the disparity between the extreme poverty of the shanty town compared to the majestic style of the city.

We enjoyed an excellent dinner in the hotel and were taken to a nightclub with a couple of men whom we'd met almost immediately upon arrival. We didn't appreciate at the time that an evening at a nightclub was special for South African visitors, as nightclubs were not allowed in South Africa. We were soon to learn that South Africa was quite a puritanical society.

After a much-needed night's sleep, the next morning, we flew to Durban, South Africa. I had ten pounds sterling in my pocket when I left home, as well as a valid return ticket and the promise of accommodation with Penny's cousin on arrival in Pietermaritzburg. We were also confident that our physiotherapy credentials would provide ready jobs to enable us to support ourselves, although we hadn't applied for any work prior to departure.

Penny had recently bought a secondhand Mini, which she was very proud of. Her brother agreed to ship it to her from Southampton to Durban. We would then be able to travel round the country in our own vehicle. I don't think Penny realised, at this stage, that I didn't yet have a driver's licence.

On arrival at Durban Airport, on the east coast of South Africa, we were met by Penny's relatives.

"Penny, how wonderful to see you. Welcome to Africa," Rosemary said as she gave her a big hug with a beaming smile.

"Oh Rosemary, how wonderful, after all this time," Penny said. "This is my friend, Hilary."

"Welcome, Hilary," both Rosemary and her husband, Doug, replied as we also exchanged hugs.

"Hello, so pleased to meet you. Thank you for welcoming us here," I shyly replied.

Amidst exciting conversation, Doug drove us inland from this large city to Pietermaritzburg, which was to be our home for the next few weeks and our base for the duration of our stay. The luxuriant scenery along the route was of rolling hills with rich green vegetation. We tried to take in our new environs at the same time as enjoying animated conversation. Rosemary was obviously very excited to see Penny, which she reciprocated.

Rosemary and Doug, along with their three young children, lived in a secluded home with a beautiful tropical garden and a stream running through it. We were warmly welcomed into their home at Wembley Terrace. Rosemary had a bubbly personality, and her sense of humour soon became evident. Doug was a little more reserved. Rosemary's father, Uncle Ken, came over, and he also greeted us enthusiastically.

"Well, I'll go hopping backwards," he said as he gave Penny a huge hug. "Welcome to South Africa."

Penny reciprocated with a loving hug. "This is Hilary," she said.

"Welcome, Hilary. I'm going to take you both sightseeing around Pietermaritzburg tomorrow. I'll show you some of the local nature parks and some of the churches I built."

We exchanged hugs, and I said, "That will be wonderful. I am so excited to be here."

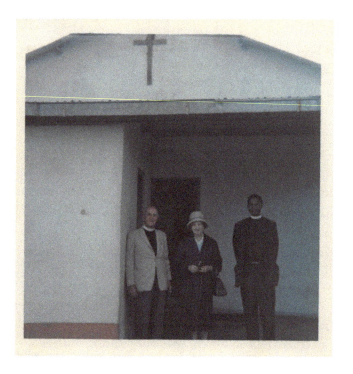

Uncle Ken, Aunt Hilda, Priest outside church

Uncle Ken was very warm and immediately accepted me as part of the family. I became endeared to him, and he became instrumental in increasing our enjoyment and understanding of the country. He lived with his sister, Hilda, not far from Rosemary and Doug's home.

Uncle Ken lost his leg as a young man in the First World War, and one of his endearing exclamations was, "Well I'll go hopping backwards!" This was, in fact, a common sight as he frequently hopped to regain his balance. Uncle Ken's father was Charles Johnson, archdeacon of Zululand, who was largely responsible for spreading Christianity and bringing healthcare to the Zulu communities. Uncle Ken was fluent in Zulu as well as English.

We enjoyed our first day and evening there, getting to know the family. Hilda also came to visit. There were three children under five: Carol, Val, and baby Peter. We gradually learnt more about the culture through conversation. Doug wanted to know if we had a copy of *Sgt. Pepper's Lonely Hearts Club Band*. The Beatles were banned in South Africa due to John Lennon's comment comparing them to Jesus. Doug was desperate to hear as much as we could tell him about them. Even the children's book *Black Beauty* was banned due to its title. This was another example of South African Puritanism and racial bias.

There was no television in South Africa in the sixties as the government didn't want to cause unrest by showing programming from the rest of the world. They also wanted to maintain the Afrikaans language. This meant that many South Africans who hadn't travelled outside their country believed that racial segregation was the norm. Our miniskirts—all the rage in England—raised eyebrows and caused comments. We obviously had much to learn.

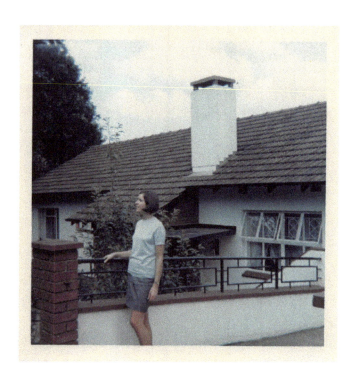

Penny at Wembley Terrace

CHAPTER 2

PIETERMARITZBURG

We woke to the sound of frogs croaking and crickets chirping as the stream gently babbled through their garden. We enjoyed a breakfast of fried mealie meal, which quickly became a favourite. Mealie meal is similar to cornmeal and is eaten extensively in parts of Africa. It can be cooked like porridge or, my preference, made more solid then fried and served as a side dish with meat.

I wandered out in the garden and was thrilled to see a troupe of monkeys swinging from the trees. There were colourful red flame trees and purple jacaranda as well as clumps of bamboo. Strelitzia, or birds of paradise, bloomed amongst the protea and salvia. Pawpaw hung from a tree, which soon became a favourite fruit. The whole garden was so colourful and tropical. It was situated in a dell below street level, and we could walk out the dining room patio doors into this peaceful oasis.

Uncle Ken came by in the morning. He cheerfully greeted us and invited us out to see the surrounding sights with him. He drove us to nearby Wylie Park, which hosted many native plants and trees of South Africa including spectacular birds of paradise as well as aloes and large areas of bamboo and bougainvillea. We also saw guava, and the red-hot pokers provided large splashes of colour. Yellow weaver birds darted in and out amongst the trees, building their nests. These are small beautiful yellow birds, which weave intricate nests from surrounding vegetation and grasses. The nests suspend from branches in the trees. Uncle Ken walked us up the trails to Worlds View, where we got a spectacular view over Pietermaritzburg and the surrounding hills.

After leaving Wylie Park, he took us out for lunch then drove us to the Lion Park on the outskirts of town. This was very exciting for us as it felt like going on safari, although the lions were actually enclosed in the park, but they were free to roam along the grassland and wooded areas. We really felt like we were in Africa now and the warmth of the sun and surrounding air were unmistakably African.

We returned to Doug and Rosemary's for supper, where they organised a braaivleis, which is Afrikaans for barbecue. They cooked boerewors, which is sausage, and mealies, corn. They invited a couple of friends over, Andre and Tony, who became frequent visitors and took us out on several trips during our stay. They and Doug enjoyed car rallies, so we ventured on one or two of them, which was like driving over dry rocky waterfalls while following clues from one point to another before winding up at a central place for another braai.

We were already settling into our new home away from home and felt embraced by this warm, friendly family. I particularly enjoyed the unusual food. Rosemary introduced me to putting cheese on my honey and toast, which I loved and continue to do to this day. Rosemary often fried gem squash sprinkled with cinnamon, particularly for breakfast, which was delicious. Another tasty meal was bobotie, a Malay concoction similar to curried meatloaf. This is still one of my favourites, but now I make it with Canadian moose meat.

After we'd been in Pietermaritzburg for a couple of days, we visited the local hospital to see if they needed any physiotherapists. Unfortunately, we found they were fully staffed. We couldn't even find jobs as shop assistants, so we rang the Addington Hospital in Durban. They were desperate for physiotherapists so we made arrangements that we would both start work there the following week. We were happy to accept six-week locums as this fit our plans perfectly for eventually travelling around the Garden Route to Cape Town. It was too far of a commute from Maritzburg, so we booked into the Howard College Residence in Durban for the weekdays so we could return to Maritzburg on weekends.

A friend of my sister's, Martin Prosser, also lived in Pietermaritzburg, so I looked him up after I'd been there a few days. He was a civil engineer and he had worked in the same office as my sister, who was a secretary in their London office. We had several mutual friends in London. He was very English and had a great sense of humour. He took me out for a wonderful lobster dinner in Durban. This was followed by a walk along the beach where we saw the lighted ships on the horizon under the southern cross and brilliant stars. Martin became a frequent visitor to Wembley Terrace. Rosemary, Doug, and Uncle Ken got along very well with him and enjoyed his company.

A couple of days later, Penny's Mini arrived by boat, so Martin drove us into Durban to pick it up. It was wonderful to now have wheels and the independence to travel as needed. The Morris Mini-Minor was a very popular car at the time. It only had two doors, but four seats. Ours was light grey in colour and looked as good as new, although it was secondhand.

Unfortunately, I didn't yet have a driver's licence, so Penny had to do all the driving, and I became the navigator. They drive on the same side of the road as in England, so that part was easy to manage. All the road signs were bilingual, so we gradually learnt some Afrikaans words such as "Hou Links": Keep Left.

The following weekend, Doug and Rosemary took us to Howick Falls on the outskirts of the city, which were quite spectacular. The Umgeni River drops three hundred feet over a rocky cliff into a broiling pool below. We enjoyed a picnic lunch there and watched their children play in the park before walking along the hiking trails. We then continued to nearby Midmar Dam, also on the Umgeni River. There is a yacht club there, so we watched them sailing while we wandered along the shore.

On the Sunday, Martin took me to communion, after which he and Uncle Ken came for a large lunch. Martin's father was a bishop in England and his brother was a monk in Rhodesia. Uncle Ken was a canon in Pietermaritzburg and Zululand and his father had been archdeacon of Zululand, so they had plenty to talk about.

Uncle Ken asked us over dinner, "Would you like to go to Zululand with me and see some of the missions we initiated?" Penny's ears and mine pricked up as we smiled broadly.

"Of course, we'd love to come," we replied. "When can we go?"

"Hopefully you'll get some time off work around Christmas, and we can go then. I have several family members there we could stay with," Uncle Ken replied.

"That would be wonderful," we said as we gave Uncle Ken a big hug.

14   PIETERMARITZBURG

This would be a great chance to see more of the country and hopefully get to meet some African families. We were excited at the prospect.

After lunch, the family took us to Queen Elizabeth Park, which is a nature reserve close to town. We saw delicate impala, which are swift-running, graceful antelope, and several zebra as we wandered through the park amidst the lush vegetation and flowering trees. Pietermaritzburg is a beautiful city with so many natural attractions close by.

Once we returned home, we made plans for our trip to Durban where we were due to start work in the morning. We had to leave Pietermaritzburg at six in the morning in order to make the one-hour drive and find our way around Durban to the Addington Hospital and to the hostel where we would stay during the week.

CHAPTER 3

ARRIVAL IN DURBAN

We arrived in Durban, squinting into the rising sun as we drove. Addington Hospital was easy to find as it is a large building right on the Indian ocean. Howard House, our hostel, was perched on a hill nearby, and we drove there first to unload our luggage and change into our white lab coat uniforms. We were delighted to find that we had a balcony overlooking the harbour in adjacent rooms. After we'd changed, we walked down through gardens to the hospital and found the physiotherapy department on the ground floor.

There we met Dr Schultze, who gave us our assignments. I was to work on the medical wards in the morning then in the gym and hydrotherapy pool in the afternoon. One of the staff gave us an orientation to the layout of the hospital. This was a European hospital, so all the staff and patients were White. This was our first introduction to the system of Apartheid.

After our orientation, we had a full hour for our lunch break. We couldn't believe our luck and immediately crossed the main road to the beach. This was amazing. The sand was pure white but so hot. We took a few steps before exclaiming, "Ouch!"

and hurriedly put our sandals back on to walk on the scorching hot sand. This was midday and the sun shone relentlessly. It didn't take us long to learn that you could easily burn in just half an hour. We ran into the surf and relished in its coolness. The Indian Ocean is warm but not nearly as hot as the sandy beach. We soon got in the habit of enjoying our lunch breaks on the beach but were careful to cover up to prevent burning, and from then on, we always wore sandals.

I enjoyed working in the hydrotherapy pool in the afternoons. One day my first patient was a young man who had the Bends. I had never heard of this before, but it is a serious condition caused by fast change in pressure when surfacing too fast from diving. Nitrogen bubbles are released into the tissues and can cause a multitude of symptoms. If the condition isn't corrected immediately, by administering hyperbaric oxygen, the patient can die. In this case, the patient had severe joint pain and was unable to walk. Submersing himself in the warm water of the pool was therapeutic, and we could do range of motion exercises, assisted by the buoyancy of the water, without pain. After a few weeks, as he improved, he started to walk with the support of the water. With practise, this could gradually progress to ambulation on land.

Apart from interesting work in a beautiful setting, we also explored up and down the east coast. We followed up on some addresses of friends from home and visited families in these small coastal towns. We were always treated to convivial hospitality and sumptuous meals. One place we visited was Umlhanga Rocks and Umdloti beach where we had lobster dinner overlooking the Indian Ocean and the rolling surf. I thought, *Work in London never offers opportunities like this.*

Durban is a large city, with a population of approximately eight hundred thousand in 1967, and has an excellent outdoor

Indian food market, where we often shopped. There were plenty of restaurants and a variety of high-quality shops. One day we stopped for lunch at a small café, where I had a grilled cheese sandwich. I was amazed by how good it tasted, and it has since become my favourite quick, cheap lunch. I can't imagine why I had never discovered anything so simple before I turned twenty-three and travelled to South Africa.

We went back to Pietermaritzburg most weekends, but we did work Saturdays too. Friends took us for a drive to the Valley of 1,000 Hills one Sunday. This is a most beautiful area of rolling hills covered in dense green bush. On some of the hills, our vehicle overheated and the rest of us had to get out and walk or occasionally push the car up the steep dirt hills. Young African boys came running out of the bush on these occasions, smiling, and helped us push the car up the hills. The mesmerising sound of African music, drumming and singing, drifted up from the valley below. Smoke wafted up from the village cooking fires. One time we watched women dancing, totally unaware that they were being watched, but so rhythmical and natural. Many of these experiences were the essence of Africa and so evocative and memorable.

Amazingly, the hospital gave us a week off over Christmas. This was fantastic, and we made our plans to go to Zululand with Uncle Ken. Zululand is situated in northeastern Natal, between the coast and the Drakensberg, north of the Tugela River.

Uncle Ken picked us up in the morning with his car. We travelled light as it was warm, and we were only going to be away five days. We drove through the Valley of 1,000 Hills again, with spectacular views of ongoing rolling green hills with African villages interspersed in their folds. This time we were in a reliable vehicle so no need to get pushed up the hills.

We drove alongside sugarcane fields and met many trucks full of sugarcane and of wattle, which they use for building. We continued to Empangeni then to Eshowe where we stayed the night with Uncle Ken's brother.

In Eshowe, we met Bishop Zulu, the first African Bishop of Zululand. Uncle Ken conversed with him fluently in Zulu. There are lots of clicks in their language, so it is interesting to listen to. They took us to the Mission Hospital where we were given a simple lunch of soup and mealie meal and were shown around the well-kept facility.

This area is in the heart of where the Zulu wars raged. King Cetshwayo had his stronghold at Eshowe in the late 1860s. Prior to this, in the early 1800s, Shaka built up his Zulu clan to become the Zulu Nation by conquering many other clans, who had been living peacefully in Natal. These clans fled the advancing armies of Shaka, towards the Cape.

At Eshowe, we met many Africans and were shown inside their kraals, which comprise of groups of round thatch huts, called rondavels. Families proudly showed us inside their huts, which were immaculately clean with shiny mud floors. Chickens scurried around outside while goats were mostly tethered. We heard much singing wherever we went and watched some African dancing. Not many, if any, tourists saw this side of South Africa, but we were with Uncle Ken, who they all knew and respected. I loved being here, enveloped by the spirit of Africa and enjoying their warm camaraderie. This is how I had imagined African life when I was still in high school. Now I was experiencing it.

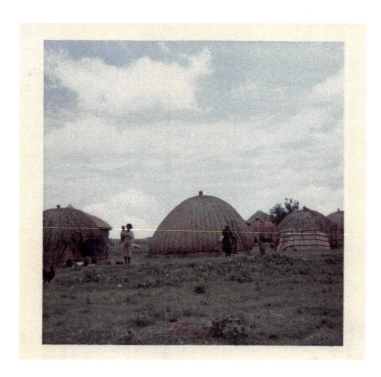

Zulu kraal

We stayed nearby with another family member and learnt much about Uncle Ken's family and how his father spent his life in this area as archdeacon of Zululand. He and his wife built many churches, schools, and hospitals in Zululand and were much loved and respected for their work. We spent a second night here then moved on to Nqutu where we saw their excellent Charles Johnson Hospital as well as St Chad's and St Augustine's missions, which were also built by Charles Johnson. During this time, Uncle Ken was working on translating the Bible into Zulu, which must have been a huge project and a great achievement.

We visited Isandlwana where we saw the battlefield from the Zulu war, where the Zulu army beat the British in 1879 in a crushing defeat. We also saw nearby Rorke's Drift, where, a little later, a small contingent of British forces defeated a much bigger contingent of Zulu warriors. In 1967, the area was peaceful, with hill summits providing pleasant views over the forested hills. We spent that night at Escort with Uncle Ken's sister, where we experienced a violent electrical storm with strong lightening flashing across the sky.

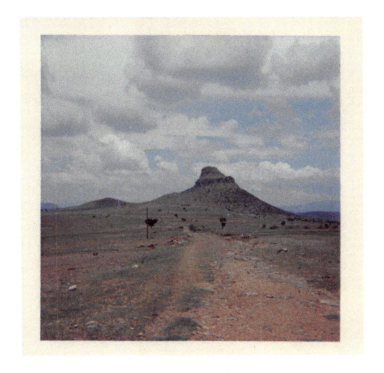

Isandlwana, Zululand

This completed our excursion, and the next day, we headed back towards Pietermaritzburg. We felt so fortunate to have had this opportunity to visit Zululand with someone who knew it so intimately. The impressions of African life affected me profoundly by opening my eyes to a much bigger life than what I had previously experienced. To the visitor, the happiness of the African people was palpable. Yet, by Western standards, they seemed to hardly have any material possessions, except their livestock and simple homes.

Back in Pietermaritzburg, there were now just two days until Christmas. We went to a carol service on Christmas Eve then opened presents and had a traditional Christmas Day despite the heat. The children excitedly opened their presents, but here there was no traditional tree. Rosemary still cooked a turkey, which we ate outside in the shade of the garden. After this, we went to a friend's house and enjoyed swimming in their pool to cool off.

In the evening, we reminisced with Uncle Ken and learnt more about the history of Zululand. He explained how his parents had come up to Zululand from Natal shortly after their marriage and how they had dedicated their lives to establishing missions and schools there. His grandfather and family emigrated from England when his father, Charles, was only seven years old. Charles was educated at Maritzburg College, so he was fluent in Zulu on arrival in Zululand, and he and his wife became much respected members of the community. They raised their family in Zululand, which explained how Uncle Ken knew it so intimately and spoke Zulu so fluently.

The day after Boxing Day, we drove back to Durban to work, having enjoyed being immersed in experiences in Zululand and beyond. The young man with the Bends was gradually improving but slowly. I continued to work mornings on the wards and afternoons in hydrotherapy, while Penny worked in the gym. We had a rich social life in Durban as everyone was so friendly.

We met some friends at a party who suggested we go to Glenmore Beach for New Years weekend, so we travelled with them down the coast towards Port Edward. We travelled through coastal communities such as Margate and Ramsgate, names which can also be found on the east coast of England, so may have been populated from there. The east coast of South Africa on the Indian Ocean with its tropical beaches, however, cannot be compared to the cold, flat seaside resorts of the east coast of England.

We continued to Glenmore Beach, just north of Port Edward, a distance of 125 miles. This is where we spent the weekend. The beach was spectacular with rolling surf on long stretches of white sand. We went for long walks on the beach and watched others surfing the big waves. All these beaches had signs reading 'nie-blankes verbode,' which means non-Whites forbidden. Even the post office and other government build-ings had separate entrances for Whites and non-Whites. Public transport was also separated by skin colour. All public benches were signed 'slegs blankes,' meaning Whites Only. This was disturbing but accepted as normal by the White population.

In the evening, we drove to Transkei Bridge, which is the border between Natal and the Transkei. Transkei was the first African State within South Africa, called a Bantustan. It was the homeland of the Xhosa people. We saw a group of young boys alongside the road, painted with white designs on their bodies. They quickly disappeared into the bush. They were undergoing circumcision rites, which is an important part of the Xhosa culture. The splashes of white are made from white mud smeared over their bodies.

After this interesting interlude, we returned to Glenmore Beach and brought in the New Year in style. It was getting pro-gressively hotter but was still very pleasant. The White South Africans always chose the shade to protect their skin, but I was happy to be getting very brown already. We were treated to a roast chicken dinner on New Years Day with champagne. After this, we enjoyed another swim in the ocean before travelling back up to Durban. As we were getting closer to Durban, our engine started boiling over.

"Oh no," said Penny. "Look at the steam." Almost as soon as we pulled the Mini over and opened the hood, a couple of guys stopped to help.

"What's up?" they said. "It looks like you've overheated."

"Yes," we said. "We're on our way back to Durban."

"Look at this," they said. "The fanbelt has broken. Do you have a spare one?"

"No," we said. "What can we do?"

"Hop in. We can drive you to Durban to get a new one, then we'll bring you back here and fix it for you."

"Okay," we said. "That would be wonderful. Thank you so much."

Wherever we went, people were so kind. After they fixed our fanbelt, they suggested we should carry spare pantyhose with us so we could fix it temporarily if it happened again. We thanked them profusely and continued to Durban.

We still had another two weeks of work at Addington before an anticipated trip to Lesotho and the Drakensberg mountains. We wanted to make sure we saw as much of Natal as possible before moving on to the Cape. Our plan was always to work our way around the country, working long enough to earn enough money to move on to the next place. I had long since abandoned my plan to become a missionary but still wanted to see as much of South Africa as I could.

CHAPTER 4

LESOTHO AND THE DRAKENSBERG

After completing our final two weeks at the Addington in Durban, we packed up and left the hospital and excellent residence. We headed towards Lesotho, through Escort to Ladysmith and on to Maseru. Penny had a physio friend, Theresa, working for International Voluntary Services at the Government Hospital in Maseru, who we were going to stay with.

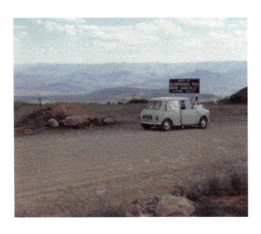

Mini on Olivershoek Pass, Drakensberg

Lesotho is a high altitude, mountainous country surrounded by South Africa. The whole country is entirely above five thousand feet and is considered to be the roof of Africa. It is a constitutional monarchy. Lesotho used to be under British rule as a protectorate called Basutoland. In 1966, it gained its independence and became Lesotho. It is a small country with a pastoral landscape of scattered kraals with herd boys watching over the cattle, sheep, and goats. The main crops grown are sorghum and maize, which they call mealies.

Being high in the mountains, Lesotho is endowed with the headwaters of several rivers including the great Orange River. This is an important asset since Lesotho is completely surrounded by South Africa, which is a much bigger and more powerful country, but it is largely dependent on Lesotho for its water supply. Since we were there, an important hydroelectric project has been built, which means that Lesotho is now self-sufficient in electricity and sells water and hydro to South Africa, boosting its economy.

We spent the weekend in the capital, Maseru, staying at the Government Hospital with Theresa. One day we drove east then went on a long walk and climbed Thabo Bosiu, which is the high point on the plateau in Lesotho. It is shaped like the Basotho hat, which was designed from the shape of the mountain. We saw King Moshoeshoe I's grave as well as graves of other chiefs. King Moshoeshoe I was the founder and first King of Basutoland. He chose Thabo Bosiu as his fortress, and he successfully defended this stronghold from all invaders, both Zulu and Boers. King Moshoeshoe II became King of Lesotho in 1966 when the country gained independence from Britain and became a constitutional monarchy. This was just a year before we arrived there. We learnt about the practice of ritual murder to take organs from living people in certain healing practices. This was an understandably much feared practice by the Sotho people.

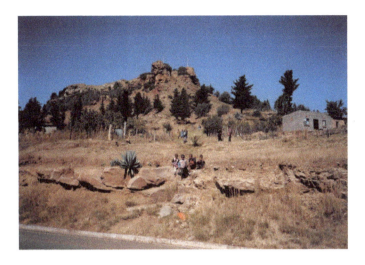

Thaba Bosiu, Lesotho

After this interesting excursion, we returned to Maseru and visited a craft shop, where I bought a Basotho hat. This was intricately woven by the local Sotho as one of their traditional crafts. I still wear it to this day to protect the face from strong sunlight. Many of the people we saw wore the traditional Basotho blanket, which they wear year-round despite the heat. These blankets are made of wool with bold designs in various colours. I now have one of these as a bedspread on my bed at home. We spent the evening at the Government Hospital visiting with Theresa and some of the doctors. It was refreshing to be away from the oppression of Apartheid here and be able to mix freely with the Black African staff.

The following morning, we left Maseru and drove through the mountains back into South Africa. We had booked a few nights at Royal Natal National Park in the Drakensberg. It took seven hours of driving through wooded and mountainous scenery to reach there early evening. On this road, as on many others on our travels, we rolled up the windows every time we met another vehicle to avoid inhaling the clouds of red dust into our Mini. Many of the minor roads were dirt or, at best, had two strips of tarmac, which caused you to veer off every time you met or passed another vehicle. We rarely passed anyone.

We set up our tent next to the stream and cooked steak supper over our camp stove, surrounded by magnificent mountain scenery. The next morning, we walked several miles up to Gudu Falls, which was an enjoyable hike with spectacular views of the escarpment of the Amphitheatre and Sentinel peak spread out ahead of us. In the afternoon, we noticed a herd of eland grazing on the hills above as we returned towards camp. We swam in the river to cool off along the way. That evening we enjoyed camaraderie with our camping neighbours and learnt more about opportunities for hiking and camping.

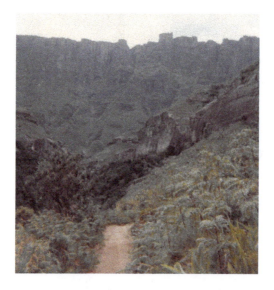

Hike to Amphitheatre, Drakensberg

We rose early the following morning and were greeted by a spectacular pink glow on the Amphitheatre and surrounding mountains. We embarked on a long hike to the top of Mount Aux Sources, a high point in the South African Drakensberg at eleven thousand feet. We joined another couple for this hike, along with an African guide, and had a pack horse for our sleeping bags and food. It was a fourteen-mile climb and took us eight hours to reach the top. We saw several baboons cavorting above us as we walked. It was boiling hot and a hard slog. We weren't experienced hikers, so were wearing flip-flop sandals and carried no water. George, our guide, was barefoot. As soon as we came to rivers, we plunged into them and drank as much as we could. After one river, around eleven o'clock, the guide spoke to us, but we couldn't understand him. It turned out he was telling us that this was the last water. We still had another four hours of hiking. At one point we passed a cave, and I was all for lying down right there as felt I couldn't go any further.

"I think I'll stay here," I gasped. "I've had it. I'll never make it to the top."

Penny persuaded me. "Come on," she said. "You can make it. We can't leave you here, and we're already over halfway. You can't turn back now."

"Oh my God," I said. "I never thought it would be this hard. I've done lots of hiking but have never climbed a mountain before. Okay, if you think I can make it, I'll try."

I reluctantly left the cave and followed the others, but this was gruelling. We saw a few monkeys and some buck during the hike. We also saw a huge eagle very close to us, which I worried might pick me right off the mountain. After several hours of hiking, we reached a high plateau, which, in fact, was the elevation of Lesotho, but we had been climbing for hours from the South African side.

A little later we reached a chain ladder going up a sheer rock face. This was a welcome change, and in no time, we reached the large plateau on top. Here I ran to the river, gulped the refreshing and much needed liquid, and flopped down on the grass.

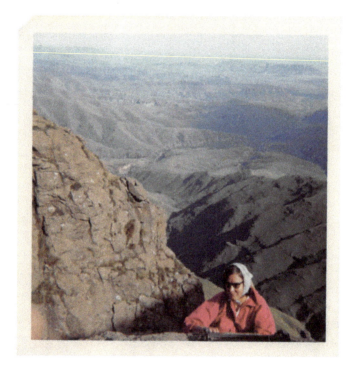

Penny on top of chain ladder

There was a stone hut on the plateau, and this is where we spent the night. We'd brought hotdogs and canned corn up the mountain, but I couldn't be bothered to cook them so ate them cold, ravenously. We collected more pristine water from the river to quench our thirst. After our refreshments, we were somewhat revived and went for a short walk across the plateau. Before retiring for the night, we were treated to a magnificent starlit sky with the Southern Cross shining brightly over us.

This had been a gruelling hike, but the views from the top were extensive and spectacular. We were above the Amphitheatre, which cradles the headwaters of the Tugela River, as it tumbles down from the plateau in a high waterfall. The Amphitheatre is bordered by the Sentinel on one end, which is where we were situated, and another high point of Mount Aux Sources on the other end. We felt on top of the world with a great sense of achievement. We overlooked rolling forested hills far below us with more sheer rocky escarpment to the east and west.

We spent a cold night on top, sleeping on the stone floor. By morning I felt recovered. We rose early and after coffee and a simple breakfast of porridge, we started the descent. Descending the chain ladder was scarier than climbing it. At the bottom of the ladder, George had to catch the packhorse, which had taken off during the night.

It took us six hours to return to camp, a much easier descent than yesterday's climb. We were happy to return to base and enjoyed cooling off by swimming in the river. Again, we had a pleasant evening with our camping neighbours and cooked our boerewors meal together.

We woke to more glorious views with the sun lighting up the mountains. This day we hiked up the Tugela River for seven miles to the gorge. The route took us past the Policeman's Helmet high above us. This was a beautiful hike and involved rock hopping along the river up into the base of the Amphitheatre. We saw more baboons and antelope as we hiked and revelled in the stunning Drakensberg. We enjoyed a picnic lunch at the gorge then continued rock hopping and

MINI SAGA IN SOUTH AFRICA   31

negotiating further upstream. This culminated in climbing two chain ladders until we were rewarded with fine views of the high falls tumbling down the escarpment. After drinking this in, we then had to trickily descend the ladders before rock hopping our way back down the river. We occasionally sat on the sun-warmed rocks to admire the magnificent mountains before returning to camp for another swim.

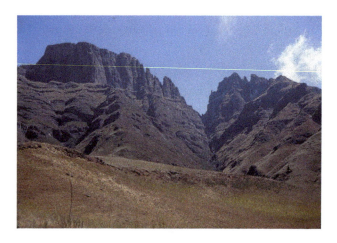

Drakensberg

In the morning, we drove back to Pietermaritzburg. That night, Martin threw a party for about thirty people to meet his brother, Hugh, who was visiting from Rhodesia. Hugh was a monk with the Community of the Resurrection, and he invited us to visit his monastery at Penhalonga when we travelled to Rhodesia, which we thought could be an interesting experience. Hugh and Martin were sons of the late Bishop of Burnley in Lancashire. Father Trevor Huddleston was also a member of the Community of the Resurrection, so he and Hugh would certainly have heard of each other, but whether they had actually met, I don't know.

We just had a few days left in Pietermaritzburg. We spent the time preparing the car, which needed a new tailpipe from all the rough road driving we had just done. We had mostly been on dirt roads, which were more like narrow tracks. We packed up our bags and prepared to leave.

Rosemary invited Uncle Ken, Aunt Hilda, Martin, and Andre and Tony, who we'd seen a lot of while we were there, for a farewell meal. It was hard to believe we had been there two months already, and we were very sad to leave. We had many people to thank for the amazing experiences we had enjoyed, but above all, it was Uncle Ken who had made our visit so epic and interesting. We enjoyed more stimulating conversations and bade our farewells. In the morning, we would start our drive along the Garden Route to Cape Town and further adventures.

CHAPTER 5

APARTHEID

*B*efore recounting the next stage of our adventures, I thought I should comment on South African politics in the 1960s.

I loved everything about South Africa except its politics. The climate, vegetation, wildlife, and natural environment are fantastic: both the dramatic coastline as well as the spectacular mountains. Opportunities for outdoor recreation are endless and the people are so hospitable. White South Africans, who we met, were willing to talk about their politics. Those who hadn't travelled outside South Africa were totally unaware that the rest of the world can live in harmony and didn't have laws enforcing racial segregation.

The Nationalist Party gained power in South Africa by winning the election in 1948. They implemented Apartheid and mobilised Afrikanerdom in the country. In 1961, they left the British Commonwealth, as they refused to allow the Black vote, and became the Republic of South Africa. Afrikaners are descended from Dutch immigrants. Afrikanerdom is Afrikaner nationalism based on pride in their language, culture, Calvinism, and a strong sense of heritage as pioneers.

Apartheid is the doctrine of separate development of the races by colour. The races were divided as Whites, Blacks, and Coloureds. Coloureds were largely those of mixed race known as Cape Coloureds of Huguenot and Malay descent. Indians and Asians were also classified in this system of Apartheid. Indians were classified as non-Whites, but Japanese were counted as honorary Whites. Chinese were originally also counted as non-Whites, together with Indians, but in the eighties became accepted as honorary Whites. It is sad that Apartheid was allowed to continue in South Africa from 1948–1994. It was too comfortable for the White South African Christians to mount any serious opposition to this philosophy.

There were White people who stood out as activists, standing up to the government against this issue. These individuals spread the word through international media of how unjust the government was towards the African people. Eventually, it was in large part the ostracization of the system of Apartheid through journalism that brought its downfall. This led to various boycotts and economic sanctions of oil, which was one commodity not available in the country. Black activism and sabotage eventually led to universal suffrage, but not for nearly half a century.

Many colonial countries are still racist but are not nearly as unjust as the system of Apartheid was in South Africa. At the time of our visit, there was no television in South Africa. The government ensured that South Africans, both White and Black, would not be influenced by outside forces with more liberal political views, so they banned television. It was not introduced until 1976 and then was strictly controlled by the government. Of course, the internet was not available at this time. Censorship was widely enforced.

When I was still in high school at St Margaret's, Father Trevor Huddleston had preached the Sunday service one day. His sermon had been about the turmoil in South Africa. He had lived in Sophiatown, an African township outside of Johannesburg, for twelve years. He had related stories of his work teaching African children and how the government had brought in a Bantu Education Act disallowing African children to attend these mission schools. He had told us about teaching these children music and how Louis Armstrong had donated a trumpet, and they had started a jazz band. In fact, Hugh Masekela had been the proud recipient of that trumpet, and he became a well-known musician globally.

Father Huddleston taught us the importance of enriching these children's lives so they would strive for future success. He explained the importance of ensuring children had enough to eat so they had energy for their studies. He asked us to reflect on our lives and compare them with the difficulties of African children in South Africa.

He made a great impression on me in those early years. I even decided I wanted to become a missionary. This didn't happen, but I have thought about him often. I recently read his book, *Naught for your Comfort*, and have learnt how outspoken and active he was against Apartheid. Archbishop Desmond Tutu stated that he did more to fight against Apartheid than any other White man. Both Desmond Tutu and Nelson Mandela spoke highly of him at his funeral. He was, indeed, a remarkable man. He wrote many letters and articles that described the horrors of Apartheid. Foreign journalists published these articles, which led to outrage from the wider world and promotion of sanctions against the South African government.

One of the most effective forms of sanctions was disallowing South Africa to compete in international sports, because they only allowed White players on their teams. Rugby and cricket were of paramount importance to South Africa, so this hurt them greatly. The Afrikaner population were staunch rugby supporters whereas the English South Africans were the main cricketers. Many of the cricketers tried to include Coloured players on their teams and strongly argued for their inclusion but were disallowed by the predominantly Afrikaner government.

Although I totally disagreed with Apartheid and joined the Progressive Party and attended some of their meetings, I never actively resisted Apartheid. If it hadn't been for the politics of Apartheid, I may have been tempted to stay in South Africa, but I knew I couldn't live under a system of enforced racial segregation.

It is important to remember that several White South Africans stood up and spoke out against the injustices of Apartheid. One such group was the Black Sash Movement. They were a group of White women who first gathered in 1956 to oppose the Senate Bill that would enlarge the Senate and enable them to win the vote to remove "Coloured" people from the electoral roll. This movement grew and strengthened and continued to peacefully oppose Apartheid at every opportunity and bore witness to each law and event.

Of course, the African National Congress (ANC), and Pan Africanist Congress (PAC), as well as many individual Black Africans vociferously opposed Apartheid, but these organisations were banned, and many dissidents were jailed.

A major difference between South Africa and other colonial countries in the sixties was that Whites were in the minority in South Africa whereas they were in the majority in other countries, such as Canada, New Zealand, and Australia, who are still guilty of racial injustice against Indigenous peoples. All these countries spoke out against Apartheid but didn't recognise their own subjugation of racial minorities.

Brian Mulroney, when he was Prime Minister of Canada, was one of the most vociferous opponents of Apartheid and a strong proponent of sanctions against South Africa. However, the Canadian government seemed to turn a blind eye to the racial injustices against their own Indigenous population. This idiosyncrasy was brought to my attention by a White South African immigrant who was perturbed by the racial inequities he found in Canada.

Another important aspect of these colonial differences is that the Dutch Reformed Church sanctioned Apartheid, but all the other Christian churches in South Africa spoke out against it and tried to improve the situation. In Canada, all the Christian churches were involved in trying to eradicate Indigenous language and culture.

Nelson Mandela was imprisoned on Robben Island during the time I was in South Africa. We were aware of him and aware of the ANC, but White South African rule was so entrenched that most White people thought the ANC and Mandela were dangerous. The government called anti-Apartheid activists, communists. We would later find that this fear was more obvious in Johannesburg. In that city, many Whites carried a gun in their car and kept their windows locked and barred. We were advised not to walk at night, which we did anyway without incident.

Author Alan Paton was also an important figure against Apartheid. I actually hitched a ride with him when I was travelling in Rhodesia, but I hadn't heard of him then and didn't know who he was until I read his book *Cry the Beloved Country.* He was also a friend of Father Trevor Huddleston, and they had great respect for each other.

I never met any of the African activists, but there were many of them, such as Steve Biko, Oliver Tambo, Walter Sisulu, and, of course, Nelson Mandela.

In 1960, the Sharpeville Massacre took place in the Transvaal. This was in response to an African uprising against the pass laws, which were instituted in the 1950s to prevent Black Africans from living in White areas and to only allow them to move between their work and home. Seven thousand protesters marched towards the police station in a peaceful protest, but as they neared the fence, the police opened fire on them, killing sixty-nine adults and children and injuring many more. This incident incited massive unrest and drew strong disapproval from the rest of the world.

This event led to Nelson Mandela moving away from his doctrine of non-violence. He started and led the military wing of the ANC, called uMkhonto we Sizwe. Translated this means 'Spear of the Nation.' He hoped that this transition would have more success in fighting against the repressive regime in South Africa. This group went underground and initiated bouts of guerrilla warfare. They were inexperienced at this, so they took training in Angola. Over time, they bombed several military and government installations. Mandela, who was a lawyer, took on a disguise with a beard and often wore overalls, posing as a workman to avoid recognition from the security police.

In 1962, only two years after the initiation of uMkhonto we Sizwe, Mandela was captured close to Howick Falls in Natal. He was driving with a gun between his legs, so he knew he was done when the security police sped in front of him and blocked his vehicle. This capture led to his imprisonment and later incarceration on Robben Island. UMkhonto we Sizwe continued their guerilla activities as the military wing of the ANC until they disbanded in 1990.

The injustice of Apartheid ensured that all the hard labour in the mines and elsewhere was done by Africans at very low wages. They weren't allowed to live in the city so stayed in camps away from their families. The pass laws prevented their families from moving into camp and the workers from living with their families in the city.

These policies together with the Bantu Education Act, which prevented African children from attending mission schools, was a major cause of crime. There were not enough opportunities for African children to attend school and get an education. This led to idle time and turning to criminal gangs to supplement their meagre resources.

Apartheid lasted until 1994. Secret negotiations took place between President FW De Klerk and Nelson Mandela from 1990 to 1993. This led to the release of Nelson Mandela from prison in 1991, acceptance of the ANC, and the institution of multiracial elections in 1994, when Nelson Mandela became the first Black president of post-Apartheid South Africa. This momentous occasion eventually took place with minimal violence and little blood shed.

It is hard to imagine that Mandela spent twenty-seven years in prison but was still able to emerge, pronouncing peace and cooperation in South Africa. He will be remembered as one of the great visionaries of our time, along with Mahatma Gandhi.

Gandhi spent several years in South Africa as a lawyer when he was a young man. In 1893, he was thrown off a Whites-only train in Pietermaritzburg, although he held a first-class ticket. This incident helped shape the doctrine and future life of the Mahatma. He stood up for his rights and the rights of other non-Whites through this action of non-violence. There is now a statue of him in Pietermaritzburg, commemorating this event.

We would later be travelling to Rhodesia, where politics and racial segregation would again be evident, but first, there were many more travels and adventures.

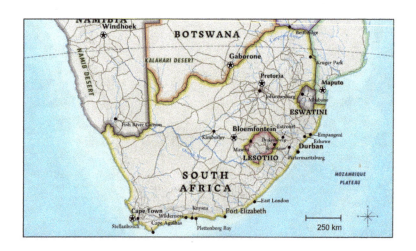

Map of South Africa, showing places visited

CHAPTER 6

NATAL TO THE CAPE VIA THE GARDEN ROUTE

We were very sad to leave our base and friends in Pietermaritzburg, but early in the morning, we embarked on the next leg of our adventure. We drove through the Transkei, which was rugged and mountainous. The population was entirely African and most of them were dressed in orange blankets and carried all kinds of loads on their heads. The Transkei, at this time, was run by the Xhosa people in that they managed their own shops, schools, and institutions but they still didn't have any say in Parliament. There was a spokesperson for the area who could make suggestions, but that was as far as their autonomy went.

We had just crossed the border after travelling through the Transkei when the car started to lurch from side to side. As soon as we pulled over, we saw that we had a flat tyre. Two guys in another vehicle stopped and helped us to jack up the car and change the tyre. We were very grateful for this help, and after travelling four hundred miles, we arrived in East London, a port on the south coast, just before the sun went

MINI SAGA IN SOUTH AFRICA   43

down. There we stayed with friends of friends. These people were staunch members of the Progressive Party, which was the only anti-Apartheid party in the country and had one MP, Helen Suzman. She founded this party in 1959 and had many supporters, but she was the sole voice in Parliament who stood up and opposed all Apartheid legislation. The ruling Nationalist Party were predominantly Afrikaners whereas the opposing United Party were predominantly English. The opposition was more liberal than the Nationalists but still supported Apartheid. We became engrossed in interesting political discussions while we were in East London, and our hosts gave us introductory letters for Helen Suzman and some other party members who we could look up when we reached Cape Town.

We spent a couple of nights there enjoying the stimulating conversation and visiting the harbour and port. We marvelled at the lovely wide beaches with rough waves from the Indian Ocean rolling in. We then drove two hundred miles through Grahamstown to Port Elizabeth, which is a major port further west along the coast. There we stayed overnight with some friends from London and visited the local sights, such as the aquarium. Again, we enjoyed the glorious sandy beaches with large surf crashing onto the shore. The next morning, we continued our journey and embarked along the famous Garden Route. We travelled through beautiful forests of stinkwood and yellowwood as well as mahogany, acacia, cypress, and the more common wattle. The stinkwood and yellowwood are magnificent hardwood trees reaching up to a high canopy. The forests were spectacular, and we came across two baboons on the road. The route took us over mountain passes and along the rugged coastline to Plettenberg Bay and Knysna, which is also densely forested.

We pitched our tent at Knysna by the lagoon, which has beautiful calm water protected from the ocean by the Knysna Heads, which are rocky bluffs. Apart from walking to the Heads, there wasn't much else to do there, so we set off again the following morning and just drove forty miles to Wilderness, which was a perfect location. We found a glorious beach with surf to play in. Here we swam, surfed, walked, and sunbathed. We met some fun people from Johannesburg as soon as we arrived there, so we set up camp next to them and even went fishing and pooled our resources for a braai.

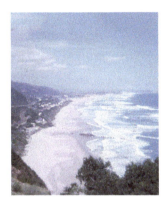

Indian Ocean

A wide river ran into the bay, so the following morning we took a boat out and rowed upstream and back. We enjoyed a pub lunch, and afterwards we listened to wonderful classical music on the piano, played by one of our beach friends who was a brilliant pianist. While we were at the pub, I used their phone to ring a friend of my cousin, who we found lived nearby. They invited us to come and visit, which we did, and we wound up spending the next two nights with them. They had a speedboat, and the next morning, they took us waterskiing before breakfast on a lake near their home. This was so peaceful as the water was flat and calm amid the scenery of surrounding bush and mountains, the best you could find anywhere. The accompanying sound of water birds completed this magical setting until our skis sliced through the water behind the hum of the motorboat, temporarily disturbing this peace.

After breakfast we drove to Oudtshoorn to visit an ostrich farm, which are largely reared for their feathers but also for biltong, which is like jerky. We even got to ride them, and sometimes they organise ostrich races. After this, we visited the nearby Cango Caves.

These caves are spectacular and were probably the highlight of this journey. They are enormous limestone caves with wonderful stalactite and stalagmite formations. They are lit up and open to the public. The entrance was a large amphitheatre with several passages that led to more widened areas. At some points, we had to crawl on our hands and knees as the ceiling was so low, and at times, we felt squeezed in from the sides too. Certainly not a place for the claustrophobic: it is, however, a most memorable experience.

On our way back to our hosts, we noticed that the car wasn't pulling very well and was making a strange noise. We took it to the garage and were told that we needed a new suspension pin for the rear wheel, which they repaired. We also needed new valves, but they couldn't do that there. We returned to Wilderness for the night. From there I phoned Auntie Eileen to let her know that we hoped to arrive in Cape Town the following day. She asked if we could find other accommodation for our first couple of nights as Auntie Daisy had a guest staying, so they didn't have room for us.

The next day, we drove the short distance to George, where they had a more extensive garage and they could replace the valves. They also told us that we needed a new cylinder head as

46   NATAL TO THE CAPE VIA THE GARDEN ROUTE

it was cracked, but we couldn't afford to fix that, so we just got the new valves. With this delay, we couldn't continue to Cape Town until noon, then we had three hundred miles to cover before reaching our destination.

Penny and I had become quite casual about money. Whoever had money on them bought whatever we needed. We managed to pay for the car repairs but really didn't have anything extra to cover any food or accommodation. We debated about what to do.

I said, "Let's just show up at my aunt's anyway. Surely they can find some floor space for us somewhere. We really don't have any spare cash, and we have no idea if there may be suitable campsites nearby."

Penny agreed, "If you think that's okay, that would be much better than camping in the city."

I was a bit hesitant as it wasn't my aunt's house. She was living with Auntie Daisy, Daisy Solomon, who wasn't a relative at all, and I hadn't yet met her. We hoped for the best and took our chances.

We travelled on and arrived at St James, a suburb of Cape Town on the Indian Ocean side of the peninsular. Penny and I were wearing our cut-off shorts and thong sandals and had been travelling and camping for a week. We walked up the path to Auntie Daisy's house and knocked on the door.

A buxom black female servant smilingly opened the door and ushered us into the dining room where my aunt, Auntie Daisy, and their elderly guest were sitting. They were all dressed in long dresses with shawls around their shoulders and were eating an assortment of fruit with a dessert knife and fork and had finger bowls in front of them! Oh my goodness, what a

MINI SAGA IN SOUTH AFRICA   47

contrast. My aunt looked embarrassed to see us, but Auntie Daisy greeted us graciously.

She said, "Come on in. Sophie will show you the study so you can drop your things and get washed up. Then you will need some supper."

I replied, "Thank you so much. We're sorry to intrude like this, but we really didn't have any other place to go."

Daisy said, "That's fine. You and Penny are most welcome. It'll be a treat to have you here."

Sophie showed us to the study. It had taken us a week to drive 1,332 miles from Pietermaritzburg to Cape Town. We had used twenty-nine gallons of gas and thirteen pints of oil as well as endured several repairs on the car.

After we washed and changed our clothes into more suitable attire, we returned to the dining room where the others had now finished their meal. They asked the servants to prepare us some food, so we followed them into the kitchen and watched them cook us some mealies and a big heaping of stew, which was most welcome. The servants loved having us there as we were so interested in what they were doing. There was the cook, Sophie; Peter, the chauffeur; a gardener; and a cleaning lady. We managed to learn quite a few recipes including Bobotie, which has become one of my favourites.

This was a large house overlooking False Bay, which is warmed by currents from the Indian Ocean. Penny and I stayed in the study for a week while the guest was in the spare room. We retired early that night as we felt that we had rather gatecrashed their hospitality, and once we had been fed, we were ready for bed after our long journey and car mishaps.

The following day, we walked on the beach before driving into Cape Town to look for work. There were no vacancies except one part-time job at Groote-Schuur Hospital, which is where Dr Christiaan Barnard did the first heart transplant operation. He did a second one while we were working at Addington Hospital. We both needed work, but since there was only one part-time job, Penny said, "Let's toss for it," which we did. Penny won the toss, and she made arrangements to start work the following week.

We returned to St James and made plans to visit Eileen's relatives in Malmesbury the next day. We enjoyed a swim in the ocean before supper. False Bay is so warm, it's like walking into a bathtub: very relaxing. We enjoyed a pleasant evening, chatting and reminiscing about old times. Auntie Eileen wanted to catch up on news of my parents. Gradually, we got to know Auntie Daisy, who was delightful. She was quite small but had a determined personality and was a most interesting conversationalist.

Auntie Daisy had a rich and interesting life. Her father was Saul Solomon, governor of the Cape. Her mother was Georgina Solomon, a teacher and later a suffragette. Saul was well known for his Liberal politics. He wanted multiracial legislation in South Africa and supported women's rights. He was considered a political radical by White South Africans. Daisy was born in 1882 and was raised in a Liberal home. They had many interesting guests including King Cetshwayo, King of the Zulus, as well as Prince Edward and Prince George, who went on to become King Edward VII and King George V of England.

The family moved back to England in the late 1880s due to Saul's health. Both Daisy and her mother became suffragettes and spent many years fighting for women's right to vote in the

United Kingdom. Once, Daisy and another suffragette tried to get an audience with the prime minister, Herbert Asquith, but were refused. As a result of this, they were delivered as mail, with the help of the postal service, to 10 Downing Street, bearing a stamp and address printed on their coats. On this occasion, they successfully met the prime minister.

On another occasion, Daisy again tried to attend an event with the prime minister, but she and twenty others were arrested and sent to Holloway Prison. She went on a hunger strike but was force-fed. Her name became well known across the world due to her political activism as she was arrested and imprisoned several times. In 1928, women finally won the right to vote on equal terms with men in England. Daisy returned to South Africa after the Second World War and went to live with her brother in St James. He was a high court judge in Cape Town. At age eighty-five, Daisy continued to host interesting and celebrated people in her home at St James but seldom two young travellers in their cut-offs and sandals.

CHAPTER 7

CAPE TOWN

We spent the weekend meeting various members of the duPlessis family, Eileen's relatives, who were mostly members of the Dutch Reform Church. This church believed that separate development of the races was sanctioned by God and endorsed by the Bible. They quoted passages from Genesis and Deuteronomy to support their beliefs, but this was a unique self-serving interpretation of the Bible. The Dutch Reform was the official theology of the ruling Nationalist Party, who were predominately Afrikaners.

It was interesting to visit more homes in different parts of the Cape and to witness the Afrikaner point of view in conversations. Up until this point, we had mostly been with South Africans of English descent and we could freely talk about the politics. Discussions were more difficult with the Afrikaner families, as their beliefs were as entrenched as mine but polar opposite. They were, however, always hospitable and political discussions were short-lived.

We drove around the Cape Peninsula through Simonstown to the Cape of Good Hope, at its southern tip. The peninsula is a narrow

MINI SAGA IN SOUTH AFRICA　　　51

finger of land stretching south from Cape Town. The west side of this peninsula is on the Atlantic Ocean whereas the east side borders False Bay, which is a protected inlet of the Atlantic. It is close to Cape Aghullas, which is where the warm Indian Ocean and the cold Atlantic Ocean meet. The contrast is remarkable, as False Bay is calm and warm whereas the Atlantic coastline is cold and has large rollers breaking towards the beach.

Cape Town and its closest communities are situated at the base of spectacular Table Mountain, which rises sharply 3,500 feet from sea level and stretches two miles across an expansive plateau. It supports some flora that are not found anywhere else. It derives its name from the flat top of the mountain with the occasional cloud cover, known as the tablecloth.

We spent the weekend exploring our environs. Penny started her part-time job at Groote Schuur, working mornings. I enjoyed walking on the beach and swimming at St James. I also went into Cape Town with Penny a couple of times to look for work. I finally accepted a job with *Reader's Digest* as a mail clerk. I started there the following week, but the work was routine and not very stimulating. It was good, however, to be earning some money so we could later continue our adventures. I visited Groote Schuur too and was hopeful a position would soon become available for me there.

The elderly lady who was staying with Auntie Daisy left after a couple of weeks, so we moved into the spare room, which had much more space. This lady was interesting in herself and was heavily involved in an organisation for Women Against War, which Auntie Daisy was also involved in.

We were looked after by the servants and enjoyed the excellent meals. Sophie, the cook, was quite buxom and had an infectious laugh and obviously enjoyed our interactions in the

52   CAPE TOWN

kitchen. It was also lovely to walk out of the house straight onto the beach and enjoy a swim before breakfast.

Auntie Daisy took us to a wonderful African play performed by Zulus with a lot of dancing. It was excellent and amazing to think that the actors were servants and truck drivers as it was impossible for any of them to have more satisfying work. Later in the week, we went to another play performed by Cape Coloureds, which was also excellent with beautiful singing.

After staying a few weeks at St James, we looked at a cottage near Camps Bay, closer to Cape Town. Some girls from Groote Schuur were staying there and two of them were leaving for a six-week holiday, so they were looking for a couple of others to take their place. We visited the cottage, called Rocks Edge, which was perched on the top of rocks overlooking the ocean. It even had a trail down to the water, which was like a small private beach. Behind this idyllic scene was Table Mountain.

"Let's move here," I said to Penny. "It will be better to be with people our age with no restrictions on our social life. What a wonderful location!"

"I'm glad you agree," said Penny. "I was finding it quite confining being with your aunts, although they were very kind to us. I can't believe we've found this beautiful spot!"

"Can we move in next week?" we asked the girls. "We'll let Auntie Daisy know and pack up our things."

"That will be fine," they said. "You can pay the next month's rent when we move out."

We were delighted. We felt it was a bit presumptive for us to stay with Auntie Daisy for our whole time at the Cape, where we planned to stay for four months.

I stayed at *Reader's Digest* for three weeks, during which time a two-month locum position became available at Groote Schuur. Around the same time as we moved into the cottage at Bakoven, I was offered and took this position. There was a gap of one week between these jobs, so I enjoyed swimming below Rocks Edge, getting to know our new environs, and visiting Groote Schuur to familiarise myself with the location there.

During this time off, I travelled with a friend to Cape Agullhas, which is the most southern point in South Africa. This is where the Indian Ocean meets the Atlantic and is a wild place. We camped there on the beach, which was exposed and windy. We still swam but it was very rough, so we didn't venture too far. The next day, we moved on to Hermanus, which has a beautiful beach with excellent surf. We camped under trees, protected from the wind by sand dunes. This road follows the coastline with the mountains rising steeply on the other side. It is difficult to beat South Africa for beauty and outdoor recreation, but the politics could not be tolerated. Life was wonderful for White people, but I could not settle there for the long-term as doing so would mean accepting Apartheid.

After swimming and enjoying a simple breakfast, we moved on to Paarl, which is in the heart of the wine-growing area. We camped in a vineyard and were shown the whole grape-crushing, vats, and bottling process. The owners gave us a large box of grapes, which were the best I'd ever tasted. We were just about to cook our supper when the farmer came down and invited us to their home to enjoy their meal with them. We gratefully accepted and enjoyed an amazing steak dinner with sherry and liqueurs made from their grapes. Everyone we met was so hospitable, and we met many kind and interesting South Africans.

We returned to our cottage after these few days away, and I prepared to start work at the famous Groote Schuur Hospital, which I looked forward to.

CHAPTER 8

GROOTE SCHUUR

I started work at Groote Schuur in the non-White outpatient department. This hospital was for both Whites and non-Whites, unlike the Addington, which was only for Whites. The races, however, were kept entirely separate, in their own wards. The Coloured patients were treated by Coloured nurses and doctors, so it was good that there was opportunity for more education for Cape Coloureds here. Sadly, the Coloured staff received exactly half the salary of the White staff. There hadn't been any Black or Coloured physiotherapists trained in South Africa yet, so we had the opportunity to work with all these populations.

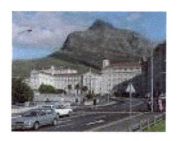

Groote Schuur Hospital

After I'd been at the hospital a couple of weeks, I was moved to the neurosurgical ward, which I really enjoyed. I also treated Dr Malan, administrator of the Cape, so an important public official. I spent a week working on Dr Christiaan Barnard's critical care unit, but unfortunately, he was away that week, so I didn't get to meet him. He did his first heart transplant surgery in 1967, shortly before we arrived in South Africa. He performed the second heart transplant a few weeks before we reached Cape Town, while we were working at the Addington. Groote Schuur was a very well-run hospital with a pleasant atmosphere. I felt fortunate to have the opportunity to work there, if only for two months. We took our turns working some weekends but didn't have any night shifts.

On our weekends off, we continued to explore more of the country. We continuously met more people who took us sailing, took us out for meals and dancing, and invited us to some wonderful parties. One fellow I met was Stephen. He was Jewish and an avid sportsman. We went to some films together but mostly met for walks on the beach and went out for meals.

One weekend, Penny and I were invited to a party in Stellenbosch in the Western Cape, which is a beautiful town sporting typical Dutch architecture. It is situated in the heart of grape country and is well known for its excellent wines. During the day, we were taken hiking in the surrounding mountains as well as fishing in the river. This party was a formal affair, so I had to borrow a long dress for the occasion. The dinner consisted of succulent steaks followed by dancing to a live jazz band and roulette tables. I met Peter at this party. He was a charming and attentive young man. He had blond hair, which fell over his face, and had quite chiselled features. Over the next few weeks, he took me sailing as well as out for dining and dancing. He even later took me home to meet his parents.

MINI SAGA IN SOUTH AFRICA

We experienced a rich and busy social life. Both Stephen and Peter became frequent visitors to Rocks Edge, but I don't think they ever showed up at the same time, which could have been embarrassing. During this time, Penny met Wolfgang, a good-looking German fellow, who took her out on several occasions.

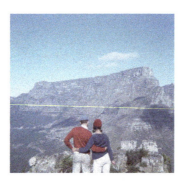

Table Mountain - Penny and Wolfgang

One day Penny and I and a couple of friends climbed Table Mountain. There is a cable car that you can take to the top, but we opted to hike. It was a hot day, and the top is over a thousand feet above sea level. Although we started hiking at eight in the morning, it was still unbearably hot. We later heard that it was the hottest day of the year. It took us three and a half hours to reach the top. We then wandered along the plateau looking over Cape Town below us and the whole Cape Peninsula stretched into the distance. We walked extensively and were amazed by the variety of plant life, including the ubiquitous protea. Some of the flora is unique to Table Mountain and is not found anywhere else. Our walking was limited by the increasing heat of the day, so after enjoying the expansive views, we started our descent. When we returned to Rocks Edge, we plunged into the icy cold sea to cool off. We could last only a few minutes in the Atlantic, unlike at St

James, which is warmed by currents from the much warmer Indian Ocean, where one can laze in the water for hours.

Many evenings we sat on the verandah overlooking the ocean while the waves crashed on the rocks below, sending spray far up in the air. We enjoyed spectacular sunsets from this vantage point, but the sun goes down very fast here, around eight in the evening.

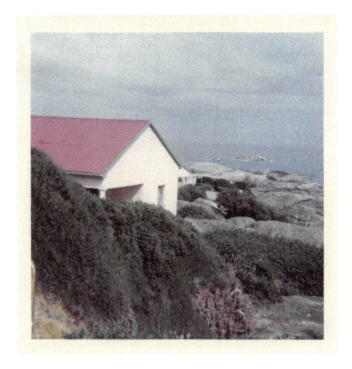

Rocks Edge

As our six weeks at Rocks Edge came to an end, we needed to find another apartment for our remaining six weeks in Cape Town. We found a good place much closer to the city, which overlooked Table Bay and was based at the foot of Table

Mountain. From the windows at the back of the house, we had an excellent view of the mountain above us.

We continued to make the most of our stay in the Cape. We both enjoyed working at the hospital and looked forward to exploring on our days off. We spent another fun weekend with eight friends whom we met during our stay. We went to Arniston, close to Cape Agullhas. This is a largely Coloured village situated at the most southern tip of the country. We set up camp on the beach and cooked an excellent meal of chops over the campfire, accompanied by locally made wine and brandy. We participated in long discussions around the campfire, mostly of a political nature, which I really enjoyed. I found myself arguing against the others, although they were mostly from England. It seemed I was the only one totally opposed to Apartheid, which surprised me.

After a comfortable night on the beach, we found that no one had remembered to bring a frying pan for breakfast. One resourceful fellow had a spade in his car, which he cleaned off thoroughly in the sea. We then had a fine breakfast of sausages, eggs, and bacon, all cooked on the spade and tasting delicious. We spent the day swimming, fishing, and walking then we drove around the surrounding countryside. This was bleak and arid but still an amazing coastline with mountains reaching up from the veldt. We then returned to Cape Town in the evening.

I looked forward to attending a meeting of the Progressive Party next week, at which Helen Suzman would be speaking. This meeting was to protest the abolition of Coloured representation in Parliament, which the Nationalist Party was about to bring in. Unfortunately, however much protest there was, nothing was likely to change. The Nationalist Party was so strong, and the United Party was a totally ineffective opposition. They agreed with many of the Nationalist ideas but were slightly more liberal. The Progressive Party was the only real opposition as they were the only party opposing Apartheid, but unfortunately, they only had one MP, Helen Suzman. They were the only legitimate Party fighting for the rights of the Coloureds and Africans in the country. The African Nationalist Congress and Pan Africanist Congress were obviously fighting against Apartheid, but they were both banned organisations.

The meeting was interesting, and Helen Suzman was a dynamic speaker, both witty and sarcastic. The meeting turned out to be orderly, but however much you protest, the Nationalists were so powerful, they could override any opposition. Apartheid became even more obvious when we reached Johannesburg, the Transvaal, and Orange Free State. Before that, we still had more exploring to do in South West Africa, Lesotho, and Swaziland.

We enjoyed our last few days in Cape Town. We visited Auntie Eileen and Auntie Daisy a few more times and they took us out to the theatre in Cape Town. I went sailing and to the theatre and out for several meals with Peter during our stay. He told me his family had a game farm bordering Kruger Park.

On one of these occasions, Peter said, "You should come and visit our game farm. Maybe after you've got settled in Jo-burg. I'm sure you would enjoy it, and it could be exciting. Do you think you can fit it in?"

"That sounds wonderful," I replied. "What do we need to bring apart from our cameras?"

Peter replied, "We'll take you hunting, so no need to bring any meat, but maybe you could round up some other groceries. There'll probably be six of us so should be lots of fun and a totally different experience for you."

Penny and I both enthused, "This is awesome! We will look forward to more adventure. Maybe in a month or two, to give us a chance to find our feet in Johannesburg and get a bit of money under our belt."

Peter replied, "Excellent! What is your address so we can make further plans."

We happily added this new venture to our list and exchanged addresses before bidding farewell to Peter.

Penny, Wolfgang, and I made plans to drive up to South West Africa, now called Namibia. This encompasses the Kalahari Desert and is home to the last remaining Bushmen, or San. We planned to take this trip after we finished work at Groote Schuur, which was imminent.

Before leaving on this trip, we visited Parliament. Parliament sits in Cape Town, but the seat of government and all the embassies are situated in Pretoria. I was delighted to see Helen Suzman in action again as the Progressive Party's one and only MP, this time speaking in Parliament. She spoke eloquently against the motion ruling that the Cape Coloureds would lose their vote, which happened in 1968. At that time, Parliament was entirely White, as the Black Africans had no vote, and although the Coloureds were allotted four MPs, they, too, were white.

After this visit to Parliament, I had a last meal with Auntie Daisy and Auntie Eileen before our departure. During dinner, we had further political discussions. Although Auntie Daisy had been most active in getting the women's vote in England, she didn't apply the same determination to universal suffrage in South Africa. She was, however, a liberal thinker. Auntie Eileen was unequivocal and supported the Afrikaner point of view and the National Party and therefore Apartheid. She was a staunch member of the Dutch Reformed Church, who found and taught passages from the Bible, which they believed supported the system of Apartheid. She went on to become a Deacon of this Church.

Penny and I packed up our apartment and prepared for our trip—this time in Wolfgang's Volkswagen. We were headed for the Kalahari.

CHAPTER 9

SOUTH WEST AFRICA

We travelled north from Cape Town in Wolfgang's Volkswagen beetle. We didn't want to subject Penny's Mini to the rough roads we knew we would encounter. Fortunately, Wolfgang was happy to take his car on this trip.

We drove through some beautiful scenery of the grape growing areas of Cedarberg before reaching Namaqualand, which is more desert-like. It is renowned for its spectacular flowers, but we were too early in the season for the main display. The road soon deteriorated into a bumpy dirt track, which rattled the car. Before the end of our first day, a rock flew through the window, shattering the windshield. We then had to drive the rest of the journey directly into the dust and wind. That first night, we camped on the side of the road on the hard ground. We secured the tent with ropes and rocks as the ground was too hard for any stakes. We put a few newspapers under our sleeping bags to provide some minimal comfort. We heard a few voices during the night and what sounded like a dog but otherwise we were not disturbed.

The next morning, we crossed the Orange River into South West Africa, which is now Namibia. The river flows from Lesotho west to the Atlantic and divides South West Africa from South Africa. We headed through the mountains to Ais-Ais hot springs, situated on the edge of the Kalahari Desert. We later discovered we were situated between the Namib Desert to the west and the Kalahari to the northeast. These springs formed extremely hot sulphur pools. We found that camping was not available there at this time, so we had to continue for another hundred miles until we found ourselves above the Fish River Canyon in rocky desert terrain. Shortly before reaching there, we saw a small group of Bushmen walking through the bush in their loincloths, not far from the edge of the road. There are very few Bushmen left now, but there are still clusters living in the Kalahari. Some consider Bushmen a derogatory term, but some of them are apparently proud of the name. San is the historical and more accepted name for this ancient tribe. We set up camp above the canyon, again having to secure the tent with ropes and rocks. We hadn't realised we were heading into such desert country so had an inadequate water supply.

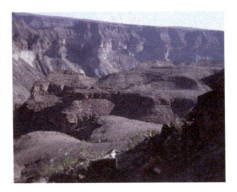

Fish River Canyon

When we woke up the next morning, we decided to hike down to the river at the bottom of Fish River Canyon to replenish our water supply. This was a 2,500-foot, steep, rocky descent. Once we got to the bottom, we lazed for a while in the scorching sun. While we were down there, we saw a large reptile in the river.

I said to Penny, "Look, there's a crocodile. We'd better get out of here."

Wolfgang replied, "That's not a crocodile. It's a large iguana."

Penny said, "Yes, I don't think it's a croc, but we've probably been down here long enough. We should collect our water and start climbing back up."

We collected a gallon of water in our large container and commenced our climb back up to the top. Fish River Canyon is said to be the second largest canyon in the world, only surpassed by the Grand Canyon of Arizona. It turns out the reptile was actually a monitor lizard.

The heat of the day and the weight of the water proved too much for us, so by the time we reached the top, we had no water left, having either drank it or tipped it out to reduce the weight. Fortunately, we had stronger liquids with us and were able to spend another night in the desert. We cooked a good dinner of steak and wine before retiring for the night.

We woke the next morning to cumulus clouds on the horizon. This unusual phenomenon expanded as we watched and turned into heavy cloud with falling temperature. This was most unusual for this area as previously, we had been surrounded by brilliant blue sky, and this was dry desert country. No sooner had we left the camp than the rain started to come down. To drive without a windshield in pelting rain and such cold temperatures was no fun. We wore all the clothes we possessed. Penny and I dove into our sleeping bags while the driver, Wolfgang, wrapped himself in Basotho blankets and covered up with our ground sheet. We all wore our dark glasses to protect our eyes from the driving rain.

We drove like this, much to the amusement of onlookers and garage attendants, through South West Africa. We stopped in at a café en-route and were given some wonderful hot soup, which helped to revive us. Eventually, we arrived back at our original campsite in the northern Cape. It was a cold and miserable night. We woke early to find heavy frost on the canvas, and we couldn't break camp quickly enough. Fortunately, by the time we reached Cedarberg again, the weather had changed for the better. We enjoyed a picnic brunch in the sunshine, removed our blankets and sleeping bags, and stripped down to beachwear. We were by a river in the mountains and spent a few hours here sunbathing and drying off.

We found some Bushmen rock paintings, dating back about five hundred years, which is very recent, as in some areas they date back thousands of years. They depicted small men and an eland painted with red dye. The Kalahari Desert is one of the few places where the Bushmen, or San, still live. They typically have a much shorter stature than other ethnic groups in the area. They are well suited to survive in this arid region because they have perfected finding ground water by sucking water up from a hole with a reed then storing it in ostrich shells.

After our refreshment in the sun, we continued to Cape Town and civilisation after a very memorable and surprisingly enjoyable holiday. We were glad to have a hot bath and wash some clothes before the next leg of our journey. We drove over and said goodbye to Auntie Eileen and Daisy and told them about our adventures in the desert. We bade sad farewells to

Wolfgang and more of our friends and within two days, left for further adventures.

CHAPTER 10

CAPE TOWN TO JOHANNESBURG VIA KIMBERLEY AND LESOTHO

We spent the next two days driving our Mini through the Karoo towards Kimberley. First, we went through the wine growing area of Paarl then over the mountainous Du Toit's Kloof Pass towards the Karoo, which is semi-desert and quite desolate. We did, however, see several springbok and some karakul sheep. These sheep are farmed and produce the wool for Persian lamb coats. We spent the first night in Beaufort West in rooms, where we cooked our supper on our camp stove. In the morning, we continued towards Kimberley, still driving through the Karoo. The landscape was hilly with scrub vegetation, but we did see plenty of springbok and some baboons and a mongoose. After a rather desolate drive, we again crossed the Orange River and left the Karoo behind us as we gradually climbed up onto the escarpment.

On arrival in Kimberley, we went to the police station to enquire about accommodation or camping sites.

"Can you tell us of a suitable place we could camp for the night or else some reasonable accommodation?" we asked the officer.

The uniformed officer smiled at us and asked where we'd come from.

"We're on our way from Cape Town to Johannesburg," we replied. "We're travelling around South Africa on a shoestring and we're not yet halfway through our time here. We're here from England for a year."

"Jah, I thought you sounded English," he said in a heavy Afrikaans accent. "Well, I'm sure you could come home with us for the night and stay with our family. We could show you some of the sights of Kimberley tomorrow."

"Well, that's very kind," we replied. "Are you sure your wife won't mind?"

"She'll be fine. Makes it interesting for her to have overseas visitors and to show you around," he said.

We accepted his offer and were happy not to have to look any further. We were now in the Orange Free State so a predominately Afrikaner population. We stayed with this family for two nights and visited the DeBeers diamond mine, which was most interesting. They showed us "the big hole" where the largest diamond was found. We saw the process of separating the diamonds from the dirt and other stones such as rubies, which are a by-product of diamond mining. We were allowed to dig for some by hand and were able to keep a few small rubies. We also watched them cut the diamonds. We met some friendly people on this tour, and they took us out for lunch and gave us tickets to the "Coon Carnival" that night. It was a revue show performed by the Cape Coloureds and was most entertaining with a variety of dancing and singing.

After our second night in Kimberley, we left for Lesotho, which was a two-hundred-mile drive southeast. Penny's physio friend, Theresa, was there, and we had previously made arrangements to spend a few days with her. On the way, we visited some salt pans. These are large expanses of shallow lakes that become covered in salt and other minerals as the water evaporates. They support diverse vegetation and birdlife, some of which are currently threatened. We also saw a Bushman nearby, who was crouching, wearing a skin with a bow and arrows. He seemed to be on his own, but there could easily have been more hidden from view by the scrub vegetation.

We travelled through Petrusburg to Bloemfontein then gradually climbed higher up the mountains to Ladybrand and finally crossed into the Kingdom of Lesotho at Maseru Bridge, where King Moshoeshoe II was now the leader. Theresa greeted us excitedly when we arrived. Theresa and Penny had trained together in England and were close friends.

We went to a party in the hospital residence our first evening there, which was wonderful. It was so refreshing to be away from Apartheid and to be able to mix so freely with the African population and enjoy dancing.

The next morning, we travelled to a Mission Hospital in northern Lesotho at Seboche. It was one hundred miles on dirt roads from Maseru, so we travelled in another vehicle as our Mini would have got lost in the potholes. The mission was in a beautiful part of the country and completely unspoilt by any tourism or outside influence. The mission was surrounded by small villages of mud huts with their donkeys and goats nearby. As we arrived, early in the morning, smoke was wafting up from the fires and we could hear distant voices, all surrounded by magnificent mountain scenery.

MINI SAGA IN SOUTH AFRICA   71

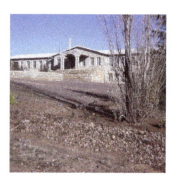

Seboche

Lesotho is entirely above five thousand feet. There were few roads, so the best means of transportation was on horseback. Basotho ponies are unshod and surefooted. They have an easy gait between a canter and a trot, known as tripling, where three hooves are off the ground at a time. We saw individual young boys watching over their herds of sheep and goats as we travelled. The boys were wrapped in their Basotho blankets and carried sticks to protect their flocks.

In the afternoon, six of us went riding on Basotho ponies. We went a good distance and were gone for three hours. I am not a rider and wound up falling off three times. The first time, my horse walked through some maize the villagers had spread out to dry in front of their huts, so Dr Kennach, who was leading our group, hit my horse on the rump and apologised to the villagers in Sesotho. The horse reared up on its hind legs and I fell off.

"I'm sorry," I said to the doctor. "I've never ridden before."

"It's okay," he said, "but I had to hit the horse so the villagers understood that it was a mistake. You'd better change horses with Penny as hers will be easier for you to control."

Penny and I then swapped horses as she was a proficient rider and mine was too wild. The next time, there wasn't really any excuse other than I was nervous, and I just seemed to slip round and fell off. The third and last time, it was beginning to get dark, so we wanted to get back in a hurry. We were cantering downhill very fast, and I fell forward right over the horse's head, ripping the seat of my trousers in the process. I wasn't very happy after that and was glad to get back safely to the mission. I was aching all over and full of bruises.

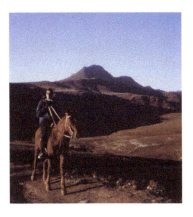

Penny on horseback

The following day, we went out riding again, this time for the whole day, and we took a picnic. I seemed to have learnt from the previous day and managed much better. We climbed up a mountain, up and over steep rocks, and did some cantering. We rode the horses as high as they could go, then we tethered them and climbed up to the top of the mountain on foot. There we had our picnic amidst a panorama of majestic mountains. Young boys grazed their sheep in the valley below. This was a wonderful day as we rode through several villages and saw women grinding maize with stones, oxen pulling ploughs, and all sorts of village life. We returned to the mission without me falling off once.

The rest of our group returned to Maseru, but Penny and I stayed an extra night at Dr Kennach's house. We returned to Maseru the following day on a local bus, which was great fun. The bus was crowded and kept stopping every few yards to pick up more passengers, some with their chickens. They all seemed to know each other and were shouting from one end of the bus to the other. There wasn't enough room for everyone, so some of them travelled on the roof.

Once we returned to Maseru, we went for a walk and found a cave with some very clear Bushmen paintings on the rocks. They were intricate artists and left their mark with distinctive pictures of hunters, often following eland. Sometimes they depicted gathering honey from beehives. We were to see more examples of these caves on our future travels. The next morning, we said goodbye to Theresa and embarked on the 270 mile journey to Johannesburg. Theresa was going to join us there in a few days for a planned trip to Swaziland.

CHAPTER 11

JOHANNESBURG TO SWAZILAND

*I*t took us over seven hours to reach Johannesburg, with a short break along the way for a picnic lunch. We found our way to Parkmore where Penny's other cousin, Rosemary's brother, lived. We arrived there in time for afternoon tea. Penny introduced me to her cousin, Loxley, known as Gobbo. He and his wife, Ginny, kindly offered to have us stay there with their family for the length of time we would be in Johannesburg. They lived about twelve miles outside the city.

It was good to get rested, washed, and fed after our travels. Again, Ginny and Gobbo welcomed us into their home with their young family. In the morning, we drove into the city, which seemed huge and busy. The mines and industry are situated to the south, so they were not evident in the city centre. There were tall skyscrapers and modern buildings. We went to the main hospital to look for work, but they didn't have anything available. We also tried a private clinic without success. This was winter in Africa and was the worst winter they'd had for years. It froze every night, and the days were bitterly cold

MINI SAGA IN SOUTH AFRICA 75

too. They even had snow in some of the neighbouring districts. Johannesburg is at a higher elevation than the coastal cities of Durban and Cape Town

After a couple of days of searching, we both managed to secure jobs at Baragwanath Hospital, which is a large 2,500-bed African Hospital for Soweto. We arranged to start a week later as we had plans to visit Swaziland and Kruger National Park over the next week or so. Theresa arrived from Maseru that evening, and the following morning, the three of us set off again in the Mini, this time for Swaziland.

Penny woke with severe tonsillitis. "Theresa, I think you'd better drive. I feel rotten," she said.

"Okay," said Theresa. "You lie down in the back and rest, and I can drive."

We drove all day and arrived in Mbabane, the capital of Swaziland, in the early evening. The dress of the Swazis was quite different from that in Lesotho. Many of the men carried a knobkerrie, a long stick with a bulbous head. They were using these as walking sticks, but they can also be used as a weapon. They mostly wore skins but many were wrapped in the traditional blankets. They looked like a proud people, holding themselves very erect. The women wore long colourful robes. We saw several busy outdoor markets where they were selling their wares, such as clay pots and beads. Our first evening there, we were invited to a party, so it was good to meet some local people. Penny still wasn't feeling well, but she managed to join us. We stayed with a friend of Theresa's, who was doing voluntary service. It was here that Theresa pulled the car door a bit too hard, and it came right off from its hinges. From then on, we tied the door onto the steering column to stop it from falling off.

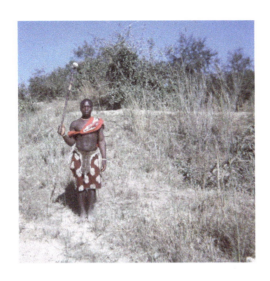

Swazi

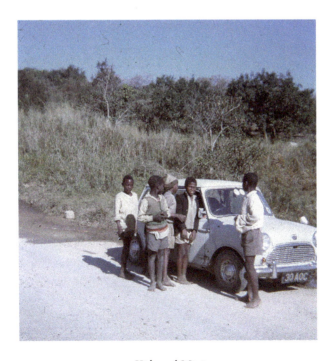

Kids and Mini

The following day, we drove across the country. Swaziland is lower in elevation and much more fertile than Lesotho. They were growing lots of sugarcane, cotton, and bananas. The houses in the towns looked modern, but the rural villages still had the typical round mud huts. Swaziland gained independence from Britain that September and now is an absolute monarchy.

In one of the towns, we met Oliver at a garage as we were filling up with petrol. He was tall and slim with brown curly hair and wandered over to our Mini and started chatting.

"Hi! Where are you guys from?" he asked. "I see you have GB plates on your car. Are you staying here in Swaziland?"

"We're just visiting here then heading to Kruger Park before returning to Johannesburg," we replied.

"Would you like to go for a coffee then maybe to the casino this evening?" he asked.

We agreed and basically got "picked up," but it was good we didn't shy away from this invitation. This chance meeting opened great opportunities for us. Oliver lived in Johannesburg and was an active member of the mountain club.

We all went out to the casino and had an enjoyable evening together.

During this encounter, Oliver suggested, "When you return to Johannesburg, we should get together and go hiking and climbing in the mountains. Our group goes out most weekends."

This sounded like a great plan as I have always enjoyed hiking although hadn't done any serious climbing yet.

We agreed saying, "Yes, that would be great. Let's meet up in the city when we return."

We exchanged phone numbers, and I wondered if this plan would actually materialise.

The next day, we left Swaziland via Piggs Peak and headed north towards Kruger National Park. Penny had recovered from her tonsillitis and was feeling back to normal. The mountainous scenery was spectacular, but the hills were too steep for our Mini, which overheated. Theresa and I got out and hitchhiked up the hill to help ease the load. We just managed to cross the border back into South Africa before it closed for the night. We camped at Barberton on the South African side of the border but still in the mountains. The following morning, we headed towards Kruger Park.

CHAPTER 12

KRUGER NATIONAL PARK

Shortly after entering the park, we saw wildebeest, zebra, giraffe, and several types of antelope. I was nervous in our Mini. The door was still tied onto the steering column so it wouldn't fall off. Tourists are warned not to get out of their car, but what do you do when your car overheats or the tailpipe falls off or the fanbelt breaks? We had already experienced all of these eventualities. My fingers were crossed as we excitedly observed the game.

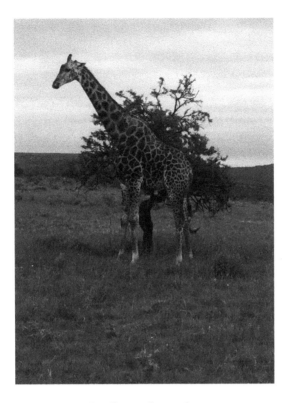

Giraffe – Andrew Roberts

We drove eighty miles into the park and camped out that first night in our tent. The camping areas are protected by thick rings of thorn bush as well as wire mesh fencing to deter the animals. We heard noises through the night, such as jackals barking and hyenas howling. On going to the bathroom in the night, I found myself face to face with a Cape buffalo with just some thorn brush and light wire fence between us. I nearly abandoned my need, but this wasn't an option, so I squatted where I was, keeping my eyes steadfastly on the buffalo. Fortunately, it didn't seem fazed by my appearance and just stood and stared, which was un-nerving.

In the morning, we packed up our tent and drove another hundred miles. The speed limit in the park is twenty-five miles per hour, but we mostly only went ten miles per hour so we could watch more game. Our excitement peaked when we saw a lion feeding on a zebra kill. We observed the animals waiting their turn nearby. The lion ate its fill then lay down in the shade. Jackals then ran in and took their share while a couple of vultures and a secretary bird came close and started tearing their share of the meat. The lion lazily allowed this to happen, but as soon as he rose to feed again, the jackals ran off and the vultures flew up into the trees, while the secretary bird strode away. The lion continued ripping and munching.

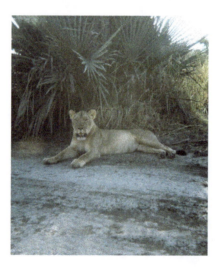

Lioness

Once the lion appeared to have satisfied his hunger, we continued on our way. We watched some giraffe feeding on tops of trees as they slowly wandered across the savanna. Next, a herd of zebra intermingled with a herd of long-maned wildebeest galloped across the veldt, overtaking our slow-moving car. Before we reached our camp, we saw plenty of antelope drinking at a waterhole, including the large, graceful eland and some smaller impala.

That night, we stayed in a rondavel, a round hut, and enjoyed a braivleis on the verandah, or stoop. The rondavel was most comfortable with beautiful yellowwood hardwood floors and a thatched roof. The windows overlooked a stream, where we watched animals come down to drink. A monkey swung in a tree on the other side of the stream, when suddenly, a leopard jumped down on it, amazingly observed from our rondavel. Life is precious but fragile for those living in these spectacular surroundings. Again, we heard animal noises during the night, but this time we were protected by the round wall of our hut.

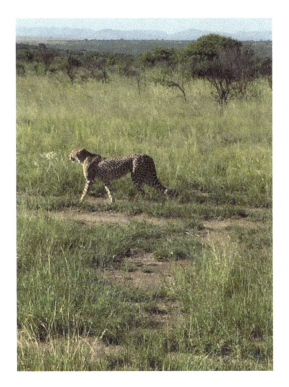

Leopard – Andrew Roberts

After breakfast the next morning, we travelled toward Letaba camp. On the way, a huge herd of elephants with calves slowly crossed the road in front of us. We counted at least thirty adults. This was a thrilling sight and we watched them for several minutes, but then we felt we were much too close to them, so decided to back up a few feet. When we looked behind us to back up, we were alarmed to see many more of them crossing directly behind us.

"Oh no, now what do we do?" we chorused.

"If just one of them decides to sit on our car, we'll all be squished," Penny said.

We had no option but to stay put while the herd continued on their way. Finally, the last one crossed, much to our relief. We could then release our collective breath and drive on. We were told before entering the park that the buffalo are the most dangerous and then the elephants, in that they are both unpredictable! Although magical, this was a nerve-racking experience.

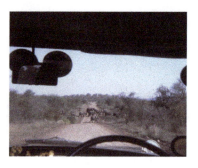

Elephant herd and Mini

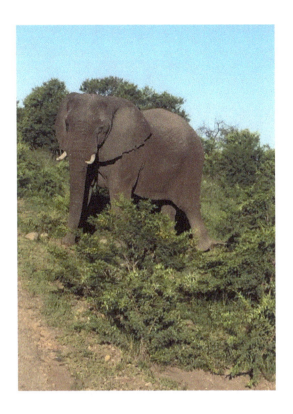

We ate lunch at the next camp and watched more game come to the watering hole. This camp was on the bank of a large sandy river and was a popular drinking place for the game. We saw more antelope, including striped kudu and hartebeest, as well as zebra come to drink.

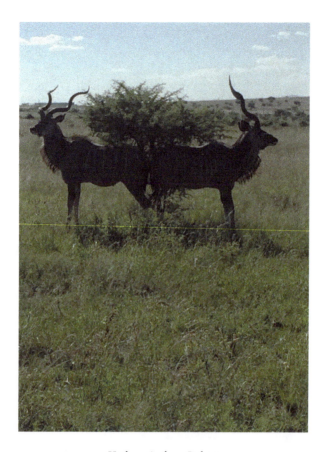

Kudu – Andrew Roberts

After enjoying these sights, we continued and had only driven nine miles from there when the water in the radiator boiled and the temperature rose alarmingly. We were not allowed to get out of the car, so we just sat there. Luckily, another vehicle soon came along, and they got out of their car and found that our water tank was completely dry and filled it up for us. We turned back to the camp, and by the time we got there, it started heating up again. We found that the water hose had perished and was leaking.

We couldn't go out any more that day, so we watched the animals coming to the river in front of the camp and saw a few hippos there. We camped here and heard hyenas howling in the night. The next morning, a fellow traveller patched our water hose for us.

We then drove out again and saw a herd of Cape buffalo, more hippos, crocodiles, and more elephants. The savanna was interesting with large baobab trees, which look as though they are growing upside down. The trunks are generally wider at the bottom with a mass of upward turning branches that resemble a rootstock. The trunks can be massively wide and efficiently store water. They produce large green seed pods, which contain cream of tartar and are rich in vitamin C. We often saw animals standing under these massive trees for shade. Acacia were also common as well as thorn trees. Closer to the rivers, the vegetation was more dense, and we saw a family of monkeys swinging from tree to tree. After enjoying these scenes, we drove back to the previous camp and slept in luxury in the rondavel again.

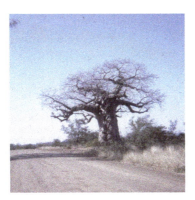

Baobab Tree

The following day, we left Kruger and drove through some luscious tropical scenery of palms and flowering trees halfway to

Johannesburg. We had planned on going the whole distance, but our water hose gave us trouble again, up another mountain pass. A fellow, who stopped when he saw us cooling off the engine, invited us back to his house for the night. He got a new water hose from a friend of his and spent a couple of hours fixing it for us. They gave us supper and we had a good night in their house enjoying their generous hospitality.

The next morning, we drove the rest of the way to Johannesburg. From there, Theresa hitchhiked back to Bloemfontein. Penny and I had two days to freshen up and prepare for starting work at Baragwaneth Hospital on Monday.

CHAPTER 13

BARAGWANATH

We drove from Parkmore to Baragwanath in time to start work there at eight o'clock. The drive took us past the entrance to Soweto, the large African township outside Johannesburg. Baragwanath mostly served the Black African population living in Soweto. The hospital was huge, 2,500 beds, and on busy days, the occupancy was two to a bed and more on the floor underneath. All the patients were Black African, and so were the nurses and some doctors. Many of the doctors and specialists were White, as were the physiotherapists as there hadn't been any Black physios trained in South Africa yet. The speech therapist was of Indian descent.

Parkmore, where we stayed, is a suburb northwest of the city, whereas Soweto and Baragwanath are situated southeast. The driving distance was twenty-five miles one way, so we allowed an hour to reach there safely. Penny and I were both to work in the outpatient children's cerebral palsy clinic, and I also worked on the orthopaedic ward and occasionally in the burn unit.

My experience in the burn unit was unforgettable. There were patients with horrendous burns, and the stench of burnt flesh was difficult. I heard terrible stories of how necklacing was a common method of torturing police informers but also was a tragic form of suicide. A tyre filled with gasoline is placed over the victim's neck then a match is struck. This is a slow, painful death as the burning tyre sears into the skin. The sight and sounds of these suffering burn patients led me to write this poem.

NECKLACING

Screams of pain
Howls of anguish
Necklacing the desperate choice
Fill a tyre with gasoline
Hang it over the neck
Light the match

Now lined up like leather
In wards reserved for burns
Fans unable to waft away
The stench of so much decay

One white face in a sea of black
Tears hidden behind their back

Baragwanath, hospital for Soweto
Mats under each bed filled head to toe
Well-qualified sisters run the place
Fluent in seven languages but barred by race

Patients, nurses, and some doctors too
Are all Bantu
Paramedics and specialists, mostly white
Believe that it is their right

To order others of darker shades
To do their bidding—just like maids

That was the time of Apartheid
Colour of skin the big divide

How is life in Soweto now?
Is there still suicide? How?
No more bulldozing teams
Can the young realize their dreams?

AIDS today the biggest scare
Virgins coveted for their care
A generation wiped away
Orphans pine for a better day

There was an African nursing sister and three other nurses under her who worked in the cerebral palsy clinic. The sister, from Soweto, was our boss, and she was fluent in seven languages but wasn't allowed a passport to travel because she was African. She was obviously well educated and ran a good program for the clinic. Every Wednesday, the White South African paediatrician came and saw some of the children who were referred to him. While he was there, all our roles reversed, as he was the boss and he treated us like bosses and the nurses as inferior. It was an obvious change, but as soon as he left the building, our roles returned to normal again.

The speech therapist was Indian, and again, racial segregation was difficult for her. She had to travel on the African buses but was usually the only non-Black African on the bus, so she felt uncomfortable on her daily travels to and from work. All the staff in the clinic got along really well together and everyone's priority was the children in our care. It was a happy atmosphere, and the children were always smiling and laughing. This was the closest I got to doing mission work in Africa.

One day I was helping Sidney, a child with cerebral palsy, to walk when he suddenly started twitching and losing control. I managed to lay him down on his side on a mat before he started having a violent seizure, which continued for nearly thirty minutes. We transferred him to one of the wards where they sedated him. He fully recovered, thankfully, and later couldn't remember anything about it, but it certainly scared us.

When one of the staff left, they put on a party at the clinic. The children played games and sang their African songs and attempted some of the tribal dances. It was a joy to see and participate with them. This work became one of my favourite jobs of all time.

The sister in charge of the clinic invited us to Soweto, which was most interesting. The small houses were similar to a low-income housing development anywhere, but they were very close together. We visited one of the schools, and the most memorable aspect of this visit was the smiling and excited children. The sound of singing emanated evocatively from the neighbourhood. It was a treat to see the happy faces. At that time, there was obviously lots of trouble in Soweto from the unjust practices of Apartheid, but this was not apparent to us on our visit. The main impression was that of beautiful happy children. This experience reminded me of Father Trevor Huddleston's sermon from when I was still in school. I was finally getting to experience and understand life in South Africa and hopefully helping these children.

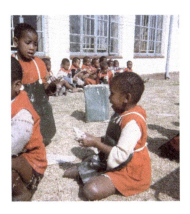

Soweto children

Another day, we took all the children from the clinic on an outing to the zoo. They were all so excited. One memorable sight was one of the African nurses pushing some children in a wheelchair with a jerrycan and toilet paper perched on her head in true African style. The children loved the outing. None of them had ever seen any of the wild animals we saw and exclaimed in wonder at the sights.

Our time in Johannesburg was not all work. In fact, we had a very busy social life. As promised, we met up with Oliver again, whom we had met in Swaziland. He introduced us to the mountain club, and our experience was enriched by many outings with them. After a few weeks with Ginny and Gobbo in Parkmore, we moved into an unfurnished apartment in the city, so we would have a shorter commute to work. This also enabled our rich social life to flourish.

CHAPTER 14

MAGALIESBERG MOUNTAINS

*T*he Magaliesberg mountains are only about an hour's drive from Johannesburg to the northwest in Eastern Transvaal. The rock is predominantly quartzite so very popular with climbers. Shortly after we returned to Johannesburg, I met up with Oliver again, and most weekends he arranged outings to the mountains. Every Wednesday night, the mountain club met, so we attended several of those meetings too and got to know a group of the climbers.

Oliver phoned and invited us to go with him on our first climbing trip that weekend. "Just bring your sleeping bag, a plate and cutlery, your wash things, and a rucksack," he said. "I'll take enough food for the three of us, and there's plenty of stream water available."

"Thanks, Oliver," I said. "That'll be great. We don't have any boots, is that okay?"

"Yes, that's fine," he said. "Just wear veldschoen or something comfortable. I'll pick you up after work on Friday around six o'clock."

"Okay, we'll be ready, and see you then," I said.

On this first trip, we were a group of eight. We started off by wading the Olifants River, which was in full flood, with our large rucksacks on our backs. This group camped in style, quite different from what I have become used to in later years in Canada. We carried a frying pan, steaks, bottles of wine, cutlery, and plates, as well as our sleeping bags.

Once we had waded across the river, we walked a short distance up the valley and camped in a beautiful gorge, right by the river. This is known as Hell's Gorge. It was sheltered by cliffs on either side so was warm enough that we didn't need a tent. We cooked our steaks over the fire followed by hot peaches and brandy, all of which was delicious. One fellow had carried in his guitar, so we sat around and sang and told stories. We found that we seldom needed a tent and just slept out under the stars instead. My only worry was snakes, so I always made sure I snuggled the sleeping bag tight around my neck.

The next morning, we went for a long walk up one side of the gorge then down the other. After this, we had to decide whether to walk for another three hours to get back to camp or take a ten-minute swim, fully clothed, through the gorge. We were all exhausted and opted for the shortest route. The water was very cold and sheer cliffs rose from either side. Once we had completed our swim and returned to camp, we were happy to have dry clothes to change into.

While we were away on this trip, Gobbo worked on our Mini. He mended the doors, secured the rear bumper, and put in new brake linings, so then we were confident we had a road-worthy car again.

Shortly after this, I received a telegram from Peter. He had made arrangements for us to visit his family's game farm next month in August, which we looked forward to. First, we would finish work at Baragwanath. The plan was to stop in at the farm on our way up to Rhodesia, now Zimbabwe.

During the week I went to another Helen Suzman meeting. She really was a remarkable woman and an excellent speaker. She had a great following, but she was still the only elected MP from the Progressive Party, which was the only non-banned anti-Apartheid party.

Another day, we got permits to attend a mine dance. This is a tribal dance in full tribal dress, which the African mine workers performed every weekend at different mines. From what we could see, the mine workers appeared happy enough and were wrapped in their Basotho blankets and were smiling and laughing.

What I did not know then, and only recently discovered while reading books by Father Trevor Huddleston and Alan Paton, is that the casual observer may not have easily understood the racial undertones behind those seemingly happy smiles.

Later in the week, Penny and I went out with Oliver and some of his friends. We went to three parties that evening, then at midnight, Oliver said, "Let's go straight to the mountains."

The original plan was to leave the next morning, but we all replied in unison, "Great idea! Let's go now."

We left Johannesburg at one in the morning and drove for an hour to the nearest place where we could leave the car. We then walked for over an hour over rocky hills and down into the valley where we were to camp. We arrived three thirty. It was beautifully warm, so again we camped out without a tent. There were a dozen others already there, and they could not believe their eyes when they woke up in the morning to find us there too.

The next day was glorious, and we spent it sunbathing and swimming. It was a beautiful place, called Dome Pools, with a river running through a series of small waterfalls with beautifully clear pools. We slid down the falls into each pool then hiked up to the top to do it again, taking respites lying on the warm, smooth rocks. Some of the group rock climbed above the pools with their ropes, but we just enjoyed the river.

These weekends were a great introduction to rock climbing as the rock was very stable and the warm, dry weather was guaranteed. We were a group of friends, so we trusted the person belaying and none of it was too difficult. We only wore our light veldtschoen, which are light walking shoes as opposed to climbing boots. A couple of the serious climbers from England wore helmets but no one else did.

The following weekend, we went back into the mountains, this time to Tonkwane. We spent a pleasant evening around the campfire. That night, we camped under a large tree and woke to dozens of eyes looking down on us from above. We had been discovered by a large group of inquisitive monkeys.

That morning, Oliver said, "Let's go rock climbing. I'll lead the group and secure the rope then Hilary comes next and an experienced climber between her and Penny then another experienced climber to bring up the rear."

"Please make sure I have the carabiner connected properly. Do we just climb one at a time?" I asked.

"Yes, I will belay you then you will belay the person below you. Once we're on top, we'll decide whether to rappel back down," he said.

This was the first time I rock climbed with ropes. I enjoyed it as I trusted the people above and below me since they were experienced and friends.

When we reached the top, Oliver said, "The best way down is to rappel. Arthur will go down first and show you how it's done, then I'll belay you while you go down."

I watched Arthur jump off from the top, holding on to the rope, and kick himself away from the rock as he descended at what looked like an alarming rate.

"I can't do that," I said. "That looks way too scary."

Oliver said, "You can do it. I won't let you fall and will keep the rope taught above you. You might even find it fun if you can relax!"

Reluctantly, I let him persuade me, and I stepped over the edge and started my descent. I didn't dare look below me but gradually started to relax as I realised that Oliver wouldn't let me get hurt, and I started kicking and swinging away from the rock as I went down. Eventually, I found it fun and exhilarating.

After we had all descended successfully, Oliver gave me a big hug and we went for a long walk before returning to the city.

"That was so much fun," I said. "Thank you for being so patient and helping me get over my fear."

"You did great," he said. "Now that you enjoy both rock climbing and rappelling, you'll have to come out with us more often. I'm sure glad we met in Swaziland!"

We squeezed hands then returned to the group and headed back to the city.

During the week, Penny and I attended a lecture on Bushman paintings at Witwatersrand University. Harold Pager gave the talk. He had been living in Ndedema Gorge in the Drakensberg near Cathedral Peak for over a year, studying Bushman art. It was a most interesting talk. Afterwards he asked if anyone in the audience would be interested in joining him in a cave for a week to see these paintings. Penny and I shot our arms up, and amazingly, as we were not university students, we were chosen to accompany him. This was planned for October, still two months away.

Another day we visited the workings of a gold mine. We descended the mine shaft to four thousand feet below ground and saw the drilling and mining as well as the different strata of rock. Afterwards we saw the surface workings, where they extract the gold. Above the mines, there are large mountains of yellow waste. All the hard labour in the mines was done by Africans at low wage. They weren't allowed to live in the city so had to stay in camps away from their families.

We were nearing the end of our time in Johannesburg. We continued to have a busy social life and enjoyed our work at Baragwanath. It was sad when it came time to say goodbye to everyone, but there was still a possibility we might return after we visited Rhodesia. Oliver put on a leaving party for us and invited many of the people from the mountain club. During my travels, I frequently remembered the promise I had

MINI SAGA IN SOUTH AFRICA   99

made to my mother not to marry and stay in South Africa, but temptations increased.

CHAPTER 15

VOORTREKKERS

*B*efore leaving on our next travels we visited the capital, Pretoria, for a day. It was a well-designed city with streets lined with purple flowering jacaranda trees. There were also beautiful hedges of flowering poinsettias.

We visited the Voortrekker monument, which is situated on a hilltop and commemorates the great Boer Trek from the Cape to the Transvaal and Orange Free State. The Cape and Natal were both under British rule. The Boers, who were of Dutch descent, wanted to get away from British rule, so they trekked north with their ox-wagons from the Cape over the Vaal and Orange Rivers and set up the republics of Transvaal and Orange Free State in the mid 1800s.

A contingency of the Voortrekkers, led by Piet Retief, decided they'd prefer to settle in Natal. They managed to find a pass over the Drakensberg where they could lead their ox-wagons and descend steeply into the lush fertile valleys of Natal.

There were some British settlers already living there, including ivory traders. They welcomed the Boers and suggested they meet with Dingane, King of the Zulus, to negotiate some

MINI SAGA IN SOUTH AFRICA   101

appropriate land for them to settle. Piet Retief did as suggested, and a small group of them headed north to Zululand and met with Dingane. Dingane greeted them and heard their request. Immediately before this, some cattle had been rustled from Dingane and his clan, so he asked Retief to find his lost cattle and return them to him, then he would consider their request for land.

Retief agreed to this and had no difficulty rounding up the lost cattle. Before returning to Dingane with the lost cattle, Piet Retief sent a message to his Voortrekkers that they should pack up and start their descent into the lush valleys of fertile Natal. Dingane was delighted to retrieve his lost cattle but resented the fact that Retief hadn't waited for his consent before sending for the rest of his Voortrekkers.

This premature influx of Boers angered King Dingane. He signed a peace treaty with Piet Retief, but then he ordered his men to massacre them and loot their cattle, horses, and guns. The few Boers who managed to escape fled down to Durban shocked and despondent.

Meanwhile, the British also sent a contingency to Natal, by boat, to support the ivory traders there. They found peaceful coexistence between the British and Afrikaner settlers in Durban, so the new British troops didn't stay long but returned to the Cape.

Eventually, the Voortrekkers, strengthened with reinforcements, returned to Zululand and this time defeated Dingane at the Battle of Blood River. They were helped in this endeavour by another Zulu force under Dingane's rival, Mpande, who eventually became King of the Zulus. Mpande honoured Piet Retief's peace agreement, following which, the Voortrekkers established the short-lived Republic of Natal and set up their

102   VOORTREKKERS

capital in Pietermaritzburg. The Boers happily established fertile farms in the area. They enjoyed peaceful coexistence with Mpande and the Zulus during this time.

As the 1800s progressed, the British and Afrikaner settlers were becoming more adversarial. The British found it difficult to acquire land in the Boer republics where they would be able to benefit from newly found gold in Transvaal. By the end of the nineteenth century, the Boer War raged between Britain and the Dutch Afrikaners. There were several different battles, which have been memorialised by various monuments erected to commemorate the victories of each side. One such monument, which we saw at Ladysmith when we were still in Natal, commemorates a significant defeat of the British forces at the siege of Ladysmith. The Boers won the First Boer War, but the British eventually defeated the Boers in 1902. These wars led to lingering animosity between the Afrikaner and English settlers. Winston Churchill was captured by Louis Botha and the Boers when he was a young war correspondent during the Second Boer War. He was travelling by train with the troops when it was ambushed near Escort in Natal. He was incarcerated in a prisoner of war camp, from which he later escaped. Louis Botha went on to become the first prime minister of the Union of South Africa.

After learning about this history and completing our tour of the Voortrekker Monument, we left Pretoria and returned to Johannesburg, prior to our next safari.

CHAPTER 16

FLOCKFIELD GAME FARM

*O*ur next adventure was to visit Peter's family's game farm on our way up to Rhodesia. Before leaving, we had to buy fourteen dozen eggs, twenty pounds of sugar, seventy-five pounds of mealie-meal, as well as several other items. Peter was already at the farm, so he needed us to do the shopping for him.

We left Johannesburg early in the morning and arrived at Peter's farm in the early evening, having driven through more beautiful country in the eastern Transvaal. The six thousand-acre farm, called Flockfield, borders Kruger Park. It comprises many species of game and, unlike in the national park, you can drive in an open Land Rover and get out and stalk the game if you wish.

"Welcome to the farm," said Peter. "How are you guys? Did you enjoy Jo'burg?"

"Hi Peter," we replied. "We had a great time in Jo'burg and spent lots of time in the mountains. Here are the groceries we bought. How many are coming?"

104   FLOCKFIELD GAME FARM

"There's just four of us for the first couple of days, but more will come to join us. Did you see any lions when you were in Kruger?"

"We saw a lion on a kill, but just the one. We saw mostly elephants and buffalo as well as different kinds of antelope," we replied.

"Well, while you're here, we'll kill an impala for lion bait and you can spend a night in the perch we've erected. You may get a good view of a lion."

"Okay," we said. "That sounds exciting! Are you sure we'll be safe?"

"You'll be fine. We'll give you a rifle as extra security."

We rose early in the morning and drove around part of the farm. Peter shot two impala, which were to feed us for the next few days. We watched Solomon, one of the servants, expertly skin the impala. We also saw many other species of antelope as well as twenty giraffe and some wildebeest. Later we walked through the bush with an African teenager as our guide, and we saw more antelope and some buffalo. Our adrenaline was flowing as we walked through the bush, keeping our eyes peeled for lions and other big game. Our teenage guide carried his gun slung over his shoulder, so we felt somewhat protected.

That night, we enjoyed fresh grilled venison for supper. In the early evening, we watched a few impala amble down the bank to the river, which ran at the bottom of the garden. The farm was in a beautiful setting with large trees and rolling hills.

The next day, we rose early again and drove around in the open-top Land Rover to see many more game. Afterwards we returned for a large breakfast, cooked for us by the three servants. Later that day, Peter shot another impala. He showed Penny how to cut its throat, before dragging it behind the vehicle to create a scent. He then suspended it from a tree. It was very hot, so the scent strengthened during the day. The plan was for Penny and me to spend the next night up a perch, opposite this tree, to watch for any lions that might be attracted by the smell of the impala.

The rest of the group from Cape Town arrived that day, and we enjoyed camaraderie over a lively supper. We had met most of the group previously when we camped with them on the south coast. There were now eight of us staying at the farm.

After a comfortable night's rest, we did more exploring, mostly by Land Rover, and saw many buck, monkeys, giraffe, zebra, and eland. We felt very lucky to have this opportunity to see so much game and to be free to explore their watering holes without any other tourists around. We returned for another delicious meal of venison cooked over the fire. We enjoyed camaraderie around the dining table before Peter escorted Penny and me to our perch for the night. The impala was still hanging there, as we had left it.

We climbed the ladder and made ourselves comfortable on a straw mat with a small pillow each. We had a gun between us, but neither of us wanted to confess that we had never used one. We had a flashlight and we tied shoelaces together and to each other so if we needed to wake the other, we wouldn't have to call out and frighten the animals away.

I couldn't sleep and was nervously aware that leopards and several other animals could easily climb trees. Nothing happened for a while, but after a few hours, I heard something padding below us then heard tearing of meat and crunching of bones below. I immediately felt for the cartridges and

106   FLOCKFIELD GAME FARM

roused Penny. We shone the flashlight only to see a pair of eyes disappearing into the bush. This happened several times, but eventually, we saw the outline of a large spotted animal but couldn't identify it. It could possibly have been a lion, but it had pinkish spots. It looked too big for a leopard, but we presumed that must have been what it was. It certainly had our adrenaline running as we felt vulnerable up in our tree. We heard it feeding several times during the night.

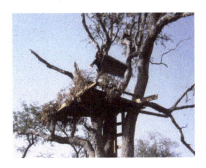

Our Perch

As night wore on, the animals increased in size and in numbers until I could see giant leopards all around us and on all the branches of our tree. Fortunately, this was only a figment of the imagination, and dawn came to find two girls unharmed. Not long after daylight, Peter returned and rescued us from our perch. We were still clutching the cartridges.

"Well, did you see anything?" asked Peter.

"Yes. A large animal with pinkish spots came several times. Was it a lion?" we excitedly answered.

"No That's just a hyena," Peter replied.

"It was quite enough for us. Can they climb trees?" we asked.

"No," he laughed. "Come on down and we'll have some breakfast."

After this eventful night and a hearty breakfast, Penny and I related our stories to the group. We had great memories to accompany us on our travels. We were then ready to pack up and leave the farm and continue our journey. This had been a unique and enjoyable experience but now it was time to say goodbye to Peter and move on towards Rhodesia.

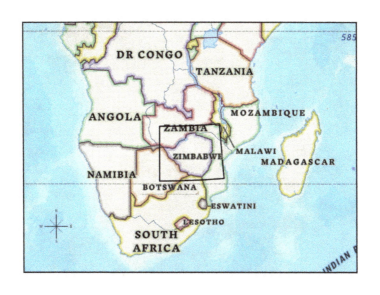

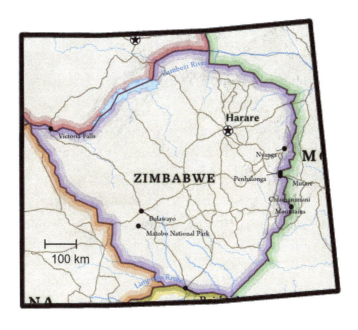

Map of Zimbabwe, showing places visited

CHAPTER 17

RHODESIA

Soon after we left the farm, we had more trouble with the Mini overheating. We stayed that night in a rondavel as it was raining through Pilgrims Rest, where we had planned to camp.

The next day, a stone flew through our windshield. Penny was all for turning back to Johannesburg, but I had my heart set on touring Rhodesia.

"We should turn back," said Penny. "The car's giving us too much trouble, and we have no assurance of work in Rhodesia. We can go back to Jo'burg or Maritzburg and stay with family."

"Oh no!" I said. "I really want to see Victoria Falls and see more of the Zambezi. Can't we get the car fixed again and hope we can find work? My aunt has friends in Salisbury we can stay with."

"If your heart is set on it, I guess we can," Penny said doubtfully. "I definitely want to go back if we can't find work though."

We hoped to get jobs in Salisbury but as yet hadn't been able to secure any. We took the Mini into the garage and had to get new valves. We decided not to fix the windshield, partly because we couldn't afford to but also the air cooled us off while we were driving as we were now in the tropics, and it was hot. The Tropic of Capricorn passes through Pietersburg, just south of the Rhodesian border.

Once the car was fixed, we continued north and camped another night before proceeding over Beit Bridge, through customs, and into Rhodesia. The Limpopo River forms this border between South Africa and Rhodesia, now Zimbabwe. Sadly, customs confiscated my Bushman bow and arrows at the border. I don't know how they could construe it as a weapon when it was so obviously a souvenir.

We drove another two hundred miles towards Bulawayo, where we camped at Matopos. This is where Cecil Rhodes' grave is situated. The next day, we walked and climbed steeply to see the grave, which is perched on top of a rocky granite landscape with a spectacular view. We continued on to see a large cave with ancient rock art. We walked sixteen miles round trip over smooth rocky terrain, but it was interesting country and we saw several colourful Matabele huts, which were quite different from the Zulu rondavels.

In the morning, we continued to Victoria Falls. Even this main road was just two tracks with dirt in the middle. We had learnt from previous trips to roll the windows up as soon as we were about to meet another vehicle to prevent the red dust from invading the car, but now we had a hole in the windshield. We saw several baboons and antelope wandering along the side of the road.

As soon as we arrived at Victoria Falls, we heard the roar and saw mist soaring above the tree canopy. We pitched our tent then walked through the rainforest and saw the magnificent falls. The falls are a mile wide and plunge down over three hundred feet. Rainbows shone in the spray as the Zambezi River plunged over the steep shelf of rocks. The falls were totally unspoilt with no buildings in sight, no guard rails, and no artificial lighting. The constant spray produces a dense rainforest where you can see mahogany, ebony, and teak growing. The air was moist and fresh as we inhaled deeply into our lungs.

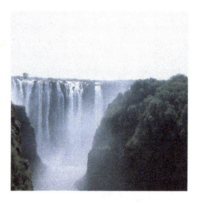

Victoria Falls

We enjoyed our supper over the campfire with the pounding roar of the falls reaching us through the trees. The next day, we had a lazy morning, walking along the river, enjoying the spectacular views, amazed that we were here on the Zambezi in the heart of Africa. We saw warthogs running along the trail, which are similar to wild pigs. We even saw elephants sauntering nearby.

We walked across Livingstone Bridge, but as soon as we got halfway across, the border guards came out with guns drawn.

"What are you doing?" they asked. "Show me your visas for Zambia."

"Er," we stammered. "We don't have visas. We just wanted to take some photos from this side."

"Go back," they barked. "You're not allowed to cross here without a visa."

We turned round sheepishly and headed back but took more photos on our way. We did get exceptional views of the falls from both sides. There are five adjoining falls: the Devil's Cataract, which is on the Rhodesian side, Main Falls, Horseshoe Falls, Rainbow Falls, and the Eastern Cataract. We had a spectacular view of the Devil's Cataract from the Zambian side.

We enjoyed another night camped among this spectacular scenery. The next day, we took a two-hour boat trip up the Zambezi River. We saw lots of game including elephants, hippo, and a white rhino. Rhodesia seemed much wilder than South Africa as these animals just roamed their natural environment. I later learnt that we were inside a large national park, but there were no signs or fences, just spectacular scenery and lots of wild animals.

We cooked our supper over the fire again that night then left in the morning for Bulawayo, where we camped the night. Bulawayo is the second largest city in Rhodesia. We got a flat tyre there, but as soon as we changed the tyre in the morning, we set off for Salisbury, three hundred miles away.

Here we stayed with the parents of a physio friend from Johannesburg. It was good to rest after so much travelling and camping. We tried to get jobs in Salisbury, but it turned out there were no physio jobs available. Penny had come round to exploring more of the country after the beauty of the falls.

MINI SAGA IN SOUTH AFRICA

We stayed a few days but decided to leave early for the Eastern Highlands and Umtali to visit Martin's brother, Hugh, who was a monk in the monastery there.

While we were still in Salisbury, we went to Parliament. This was interesting as Ian Smith was prime minister and he had declared unilateral independence, UDI, from Britain in 1965. Britain demanded black majority rule, which Ian Smith would not accept. We listened to Ian Smith and the leader of the opposition debate on the unwillingness of Britain's prime minister, Harold Wilson, to negotiate. They also debated confidence in the all-White Rhodesian Front Party, of which Ian Smith was head. The opposition gave a vote of confidence in the government, saying they were satisfied Wilson had demonstrated an unwillingness to negotiate. This resulted in no further chance of renewing any negotiations with Britain.

In Rhodesia, we found an unwillingness of the White people to discuss politics, unlike in South Africa, where we'd had many interesting discussions. The families, the ones we stayed with anyway, didn't seem to treat their servants well. The servants were poorly dressed and generally appeared unhappy.

We left Salisbury and drove to Inyanga. There we found a lovely camping spot in a pine wood. We went for a walk through the woods overlooking green rolling hills before cooking our supper and settling for the night. The next day, we went for a long walk to a ruined fort and old pit structures dating back to the iron age. The vegetation was green and lush with colourful cosmos gently swaying in the breeze. The most prominent feature was Mount Inyangani, which we decided to climb the next day. This is the highest mountain in Rhodesia but is only 8,500 feet tall.

We had a good climb up to the top of the mountain and met a young man up there whose name was Roger. Since there were only three of us on the mountain, we had a good chat and discovered that Roger was a tobacco farmer. He looked about the same age as us and was wearing khaki shorts and an open-necked shirt. He was of average height with soft brown hair and seemed shy and unthreatening.

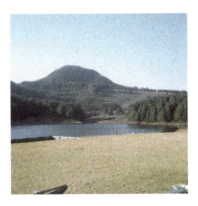

Inyanga

"After we go down, would you like to come to the Troutbeck Hotel for tea?" he asked.

This was close to our camp, so we readily agreed. It was a beautiful hotel set in lush vegetation and sported a golf course.

After tea, he said, "How about driving up to World's View next? You can see for miles from there."

"Okay," we replied. "That would be great."

Roger then drove us up to World's View, where we could appreciate the spectacular scenery over an expansive vista. Next, he took us out for a wonderful meal to the Rhodes Hotel. We were leaving the next day, but I hoped to find work in nearby Umtali, so Roger said he hoped we would meet again then.

The following morning, Penny and I left Inyanga and took the scenic route to Penhalonga, where we met Martin's brother, Hugh, and other monks at St Augustine's Mission.

Hugh welcomed us and said, "You are welcome to spend a night or two here. The Sisters will show you your rooms and the refectory where you can eat."

"Thank you, Hugh," we replied. "We just need to go into Umtali first to see if I can find work there, then we'll be back."

My memory of Penhalonga is that it was a silent monastery, and Penny and I could only speak in our room. Penny's memory, however, is different, but I don't think we could speak in the refectory or in the hallways.

Penny had decided that she would rather return to Johannesburg, but I still wanted to spend more time in these Eastern Highlands. We drove to nearby Umtali and visited the hospital. They didn't need a physio but there was a private physio who wanted to take a holiday from her clinic, and she was delighted to give me a two-week locum so she could get away. I made arrangements to return in a few days.

We spent that night at St Augustine's Mission in Penhalonga. The Sisters and Fathers at the monastery were very kind, and they showed us round the mission schools, hostels, clinics, and churches, which were all well organised. St Augustine's was run by the Community of the Resurrection, which was the same Anglican community that Father Trevor Huddleston belonged to. He and Hugh must have met each other, but I didn't realise this connection when I was there. St Augustine's School became renowned for the quality of its education for

African children, several of whom continued on to higher studies to become doctors, teachers, and other professionals. Hugh became the principal of this school and introduced the Cambridge entrance exams.

He became renowned for his principled heroism during the war of independence. The school was situated close to the Mozambique border, and the school and Hugh were frequently threatened by the Rhodesian Security Forces while the Zimbabwe National Liberation Army freedom fighters frequented the school and mission, but mostly at night to avoid detection.

After leaving Penhalonga, we travelled to the Chimanimani Mountains on the Mozambique border. The mountain scenery was exquisite, but the roads were terrible. We camped in the national park and went on a steep hike. We had more trouble with the car, which we had to get fixed before leaving the Chimanimani Mountains.

We then visited the Great Zimbabwe Ruins, which are an ancient and impressive sight. The ruins are a fine example of African architecture and building skill. They include massive circular stone buildings made of granite with thick towering walls. They are built with mortarless stone and have withstood centuries of erosion. The site, which was built between the eleventh and fifteenth centuries, covers about two hundred acres. It is the remains of an ancient Iron Age city comprising a royal palace, stone houses, and a large religious centre. After visiting this impressive complex, Penny and I parted company for a couple of weeks.

From there, Penny returned to Johannesburg in the Mini, as planned, and I hitchhiked back to Umtali with a cattle rancher to start my new job.

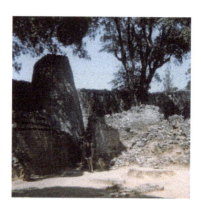

Great Zimbabwe Ruins

Umtali is the third largest city in Rhodesia but is still quite small. It is situated in beautiful mountain scenery, similar to Switzerland. The physio whose locum I was taking left me her house and servant while she was away, so I lived in luxury for a couple of weeks. It felt weird to give the servant an egg to cook for my supper, but I was living simply and that was the best I could manage. The work in the physio clinic was interesting, and I enjoyed my time there. Roger phoned me soon after I arrived in Umtali, and he took me out on several occasions. I was also invited to other people's houses for meals, which was very kind.

I worked there for two weeks, then the other physio returned and paid me handsomely. I felt very fortunate to have had this opportunity in this beautiful part of the world. Roger invited me to go with him on a road trip to Beira in Mozambique. He seemed trustworthy and was quite shy, so I thought this should be a fun trip, and I readily agreed. I was a bit hesitant about taking off with a virtual stranger into the unknown, but if you don't take risks, you may miss life's opportunities.

After completing work, Roger and I left for Beira. We stayed near the ocean and spent the day swimming and walking along the wide white sandy beach. Beira was beautiful, with long beaches overlooking the Indian Ocean, fringed with palm trees. After a couple of days, we drove to Gorongosa game reserve. We rose early for game viewing and saw four lionesses, a hippo, and lots of other game. The lions were stalking with their tails up and noses to the ground. They walked very close by us, as we watched from our beat-up Renault, before disappearing into the bush. Apparently, they use their tails as a means of communication, and when erect, they can be followed more easily through the long grass by the rest of the pride. Majestic striped eland with their curly horns and white striped flanks were plentiful, scattered over the savanna. Herds of wildebeest and zebra stampeded by us, kicking up dust. Maybe the lions were on their scent. Having savoured these special moments, we spent another night there, then it was sadly time to return to Umtali. I was very grateful to Roger for this unplanned but beautiful five days away.

"Thank you, Roger, for a great trip. I never expected to get to Gorongosa, and it was so exciting to see that pride of lions."

'I'm so glad you could come with me. I wish you didn't have to leave. Maybe we can meet up again later?" he replied. We hugged goodbye.

I hitchhiked the next day to Salisbury. I had no trouble getting a ride and enjoyed interesting conversation with Alan Paton, the author. I can't believe that this was actually Alan Paton as he was so famous, and it didn't register with me at the time, but we talked extensively about his book *Cry, the Beloved Country* while we travelled. I hadn't heard of him then, but I soon read his book and thereby gained many insights into South Africa.

I stayed a couple of nights with a family in Salisbury then got a lift down to Johannesburg after placing an ad in the local paper for a ride. It was a long journey across the border. I met up with Penny in the evening and spent the night at Ginny and Gobbo's. We enjoyed sharing our experiences, then Penny and I left the next morning and drove down to Pietermaritzburg.

CHAPTER 18

RETURN TO NATAL
AND DRAKENSBERG

We arrived in Pietermaritzburg in the afternoon, and it was delightful to see everyone again. Rosemary put on a dinner party that evening. Martin came, as did several friends whom we had met previously. It was so good to chat and exchange stories.

Martin took me to communion the next morning and came back to Rosemary's for breakfast. Uncle Ken came for lunch, and it was wonderful to see him again and tell him about our adventures.

"Well, I'll go hopping backwards," he said when we told him about being surrounded by a herd of elephants in our Mini.

"We thought we saw a crocodile in Fish River Canyon," we told him, "but it turned out it was just an iguana or monitor lizard. Our car gave us lots of trouble, but people were very helpful."

"You did well to make it back here all in one piece," he said. "We're so glad to have you back home safe."

MINI SAGA IN SOUTH AFRICA   121

We went over to Martin's in the afternoon to swim in his pool and stayed for supper there. We chatted at length about visiting Hugh and discussed our future plans. Martin planned to return to England for Christmas but then would return to Pietermaritzburg. Penny decided to stay on in South Africa until May. I was leaving for home in November on the last day my ticket was valid.

We spent the next day catching up with our mail and writing letters as well as washing all the clothes from our travels and cleaning out the dusty Mini. We enjoyed sunbathing in the garden whilst babysitting the kids and later went to Martin's for supper again.

We went to Durban the following day to shop and spent the afternoon on the beach and enjoyed swimming in the Indian Ocean again. We bought supplies for our imminent trip to the Drakensberg to visit the Bushmen caves. We visited more relatives of Penny's then returned to Pietermaritzburg. We only had one more day before it was time to leave our "home away from home." We had lunch with Uncle Ken and his sister, Aunt Hilda. We were going to miss him big time as he had been so important in giving us a base from which to understand the people of South Africa and in taking us to meet so many of his relatives and parishioners in Zululand.

Martin came for supper again, and it was sad to say our goodbyes. He had also played an important part in increasing our enjoyment of Natal. We packed up our gear, and the following morning, we tearfully left the Metcalfe family and headed towards the Drakensberg.

We drove to Ladysmith, left our Mini there, and got a ride with others up the rough road to Cathedral Peak. There we met the archaeologist, Harald Pager, and the rest of the group. There were twelve of us altogether. Cathedral Peak is a spectacular area of the Drakensberg with its snow-capped peak overlooking the folded forested mountains. We loaded our packs on our backs then steeply descended the narrow trail, bordered by proteas and aloes, to Ndedema Gorge and climbed up the other side to Poachers Cave, which was to be our home for the long weekend. This is a Bushman cave, which are shallow shelters in the sandstone rock.

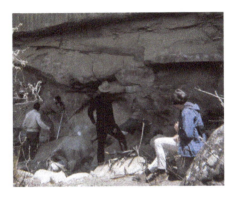

Bushman cave with Harald Pager

The Bushmen are also known as San. There are very few of them left now, having been overrun by Zulu and European intruders into their territory. They survived on hunting and foraging but only used a bow and arrow and lived entirely off the land. They are of small stature and are noticeably different from Zulu and other African tribes.

This cave was ten feet deep and eight feet high but very wide, so there was plenty of room for all of us. We cooked our suppers outside the cave, listening to the river gurgling below us. We were surrounded by high mountains, so the sun went down early and came up late, but the glistening stars were magnificent. The Southern Cross is the most prominent constellation in the southern sky. I lay on the grassy bank, away from the cave, listening to the river below and looking at the soaring mountains above, and wished I could stay there for ever. It was a magical place. It is still my "go-to" place in my dreams.

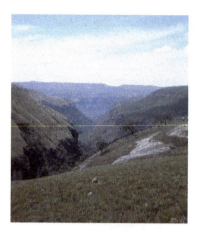

Ndedema Gorge

After breakfast the next morning, we traversed along the mountain trail through magnificent scenery with flowering proteas, ferns, and orchids along the route. The caves are situated where the sandstone rocks overhang, all at the same elevation and below the peaks. We stopped at several of these caves and saw the elaborate rock paintings. These are painted with a mixture of pulverised red rock and fat, which produces an ochre colour, and depict scenes such as men collecting honey and hunting eland with bows and arrows. They become brighter if you splash water on them, but this is discouraged, since it causes them to gradually fade.

After visiting these caves, we washed and swam in the refreshing river below. Harald Pager explained to us his studies of this art. He was a gentle soft-spoken man with weather-worn skin and a large-brimmed hat. He had been living in this cave for eight months and was writing a book on Bushman Art, specifically in Ndedema Gorge. He stayed there for two years and published his book, *Ndedema*, in 1971.

The next morning, we woke to a glorious pink glow on the surrounding peaks. We walked to Elands Cave, the largest cave in this system with more evocative paintings depicting the Bushman way of life. We continued on to Junction and more shelters with further artwork then returned to camp and enjoyed a pleasant evening with a large communal stew followed by singing accompanied by harmonicas. We walked ten miles each day so earned our appetite. We were visited by a civet cat that evening, which tried to steal some of our food, but it was quite timid so soon ran off.

We rose early the next morning, climbed back up to our vehicles, and left Cathedral Peak after a truly wonderful weekend. I'm so glad we had the temerity to raise our hands at the Witwatersrand lecture two months earlier.

We had a reasonable drive back to Johannesburg and stayed overnight with Ginny and Gobbo. After getting washed up and doing our much-needed laundry, we returned to our apartment in the city. It turned out that both Stephen and Oliver had moved into the same apartment building we were staying in. I could see I was going to have an interesting time for my last few weeks in Johannesburg.

CHAPTER 19

LEAVING SOUTH AFRICA

A couple of days after returning to Johannesburg, we were able to continue our work at Baragwanath in the paediatric clinic. They gave us a fabulous welcome back, and this has remained one of my favourite places to work. It also gave me the experience needed to do more paediatric physio once I returned to England and later in my career in Canada.

My social life became hectic, sharing evenings out with Stephen and Oliver. A friend from England, Robin Andrews, also showed up, and Martin Prosser came up from Pietermaritzburg, so life was full. Roger tried to persuade me to go back up to Rhodesia for a week, and Peter wrote several letters. Life would seem dull at home after all this!

On the weekend, we went out with Oliver and the mountain club again. We enjoyed sunny weather and did some more climbs as well as enjoyed swimming in the river. We had to cross the river on stepping stones to reach our campsite. Partway across, I was horrified to see a coiled up python on one of the stones where I had to step. After a few moments of fear, I realised the snake was dead and one of the others must have placed it there to trick us. Since I wasn't the first one to cross, I presumed it must be safe. We spent many nights over the year camping out under the stars without a tent. My only worry was the possibility of snakes, so I always made sure my sleeping bag was secured tightly around my neck before I settled for the night and fell asleep.

Meeting Oliver and getting introduced to the mountain club certainly enhanced our stay in Johannesburg. These hiking and climbing experiences strengthened my love of the outdoors and led to a lifelong love of hiking in the mountains. Two of the climbers planned on being in London over New Years, so we agreed to meet up in Aviemore in the Cairngorms in Scotland for some skiing. These same fellows had chased snow in South Africa when it snowed high up in the mountains, but I doubt they ever found anything skiable.

One day at work, Penny and I showed our slides of Kruger Park to the children at the clinic. It was wonderful as they were so excited since they had never seen anything like that before. One boy, who usually never spoke, called out the names of things he saw on the screen. This was a remarkable success. It was wonderful to see them all so happy and excited.

I left work two days before I was due to leave South Africa. Penny would stay in Johannesburg a while longer then return to Pietermaritzburg. I had one day in which to clean up and sort out my belongings. I sent several parcels home so that I wouldn't have excess baggage for the flight.

The last week I was in Johannesburg, I went out every night with various friends for meals, a concert, a folk festival, and a play. It all culminated in a farewell party of twenty people on the last day at our apartment. We then moved to a friend's house who had a pool, so we enjoyed an early morning floodlit swim. I had to leave the next morning for Lourenco Marques. Robin Andrews agreed to take me up there and spend the last few days in Africa with me before he had to return to Johannesburg.

The next morning, I hugged Penny goodbye.

"Thank you for a wonderful year," I said. "Although the Mini gave us so much trouble, we couldn't have managed without it. Make sure you write to me and keep me up to date on your plans."

"You write too," she said. "It will seem strange without you, but I'll go back to Rosemary's soon and spend more time with them. We certainly had a blast!"

It was a sad farewell as we had done so much together and we got along so well, although we were both quite different. We had worked our way around the country, but we still left our finances pretty tight. We were both casual about money and whoever had spare cash paid for what was needed. This worked out well and we were fortunate that we both had similar attitudes.

It was kind of Robin Andrews to agree to take me up to Lourenco Marques. We still had a few days before my flight, so I was hoping for good weather and some beach time. We arrived there in the early evening and went out for an excellent dinner and to a nightclub. Nightclubs and casinos were banned in South Africa, so it was a treat to partake in this entertainment.

Unfortunately, it rained for the next few days we were there, so we had lazy days but wonderful evenings of dining and dancing. One day we took a boat trip up the river and saw some hippo and crocodiles. On my last day, it was sunny and hot. We spent the morning on the beach, swimming and snorkelling, then headed for the airport. Although I had sent a large parcel home, I still had excess baggage so discarded my tennis racquet and a few other items before checking in. I still had to borrow ten pounds from Robin to pay for my overweight bag.

I had ten pounds sterling in my pocket when I left England and was minus ten pounds on leaving South Africa, but what a year we had had. I realised I would have to get back to work soon after reaching home. I was very thankful to Robin for escorting me on this last leg of my journey, and again, it was sad to say goodbye.

I flew home over Johannesburg and landed in Luanda and again in Tripoli, where it was very hot. That is where I sadly left Africa but eagerly anticipated England, family, and home. This completed a wonderful year away, where I embraced all opportunities as they arose. This philosophy has enriched my life and these experiences in South Africa were instrumental in forming my future path.

EPILOGUE

After returning to England, I started work at the Franklin Delano Roosevelt School for disabled children. This gave me school holidays, and that summer I applied as a tour guide for the British Ramblers Association. They were planning a three-week excursion to South Africa. In the application, I was asked which languages I spoke. I stated Afrikaans and Zulu, since I had learnt a few words in both of these languages and was fairly sure that no one in England could speak either one. This probably gave me an edge, and I returned to South Africa in August with eighteen Ramblers, all expenses paid.

This was a three-week excursion, one week at Kirstenbosch botanical gardens in the Cape, one week hiking at Cathedral Peak and one week safari at Hluhluwe Game Reserve in Zululand. We flew to Johannesburg, and I met up with Oliver again and spent a couple of days there with him, which we enjoyed. We took our tour to Pretoria for the day. The next day, we travelled by bus to Durban, and I met up with Penny and went with her to Pietermaritzburg to see all the family. By this time, she and Martin were engaged to be married. It was lovely to see Uncle Ken and all of them again. Penny brought me back to Durban and we arranged for the Ramblers group to visit the lion park and the Valley of 1,000 Hills, which they found very impressive.

Most of the group took the train to the Cape to see the Kirstenbosch botanical gardens while the rest of them stayed in Durban and I visited in Pietermaritzburg.

When we went to Hluhluwe, I was responsible for buying all the food for our safari, which we did at the large Indian market in Durban. Once we reached the game reserve, we had two game guides to look after the group: one White, one African, and both armed. Hluhluwe is a non-motorised game reserve for walking only, and its main specialty is white rhino. We split up into two groups: one group stalked the animals whenever we found tracks, and the other group kept away from them as they were older and less agile. At one point, when we came really close to a rhino, we had to climb up thorn trees for safety. The guide had his gun ready but didn't have to use it. We saw a lot of game on this trip, including a lion on a kill. Another time we came face to face with a black rhino, and the guide had to fire a shot in the air to scare it away. It was a wonderful safari with lots of excitement. Most of the riverbeds were dry as the rainy season was still to come, so there were large expanses of flat, wide, cracked earth. Even the Umfolozi River was very low.

After this, we went to the Drakensberg and had a wonderful week of hiking, climbing, and seeing more caves in the Cathedral Peak area. Several of the group also went pony riding. The Ramblers were very impressed with the spectacular scenery and wonderful hiking terrain. We then returned to Johannesburg for our flight home and left South Africa.

These adventures took place a long time ago. Nelson Mandela was released from prison in 1991. Multi-racial elections took place in 1994, and the ANC took over government with Nelson Mandela as their leader and president of South Africa. These were momentous changes.

I have returned to South Africa a couple of times since then. Once, my husband and I met up with Auntie Eileen in Cape Town, and my parents visited there at the same time, so we had a lovely reunion. My husband and I rented a car and we drove round the garden route to Pietermaritzburg and stayed with our friends there again. We flew from there to Kenya for a safari and on to England to see my family.

Many years later, Penny and I met in Pietermaritzburg and stayed with Rosemary, and the three of us went back to the Drakensberg for some wonderful hiking, where we stayed in Bushman caves again. This visit was after the end of Apartheid, so the difference was quite noticeable. The European families were more nervous and had bars on their windows and fences around their properties. Carjacking was quite common, so Rosemary kept her car in dilapidated shape so it would be less enticing for a carjacker.

I am amazed there hasn't been more violence considering how the government treated the Africans under Apartheid. One hears more about intertribal fighting rather than serious racial crime. Nelson Mandela must take a lot of the credit for this peaceful transition. Archbishop Desmond Tutu headed the Truth and Reconciliation hearings, which were also important in this transition of power.

Long after I left South Africa, I did pursue my dream of missionary work, not in the sense of spreading Christianity but more in volunteering my services as a physiotherapist. I spent a year teaching physiotherapy and helping to develop a community-based disability program in South India. With colleagues, we set up a charity in Canada to support this work. I continued with this project over a twenty-five year period and published a book about it, *Footsteps to Freedom – Tales of Therapy in Rural India*. The church I now attend, St Giles Presbyterian Church, supports this work as one of their missions.

I also volunteered with a medical team to Tibet under the auspices of Tulku Akong Rinpoche. There I spent much time absorbing and learning about Buddhism. I spent a couple of months volunteering as a physiotherapist with the Root Institute in Bodh Gaya, Bihar, India, which is where the Buddha attained his enlightenment under the Bodhi tree. I also volunteered physiotherapy services for a few months in Bhutan and in Ladakh, both predominantly Buddhist communities.

All of these experiences have enriched my life considerably, and I am thankful for all the influencers in my life who have encouraged me to grasp all opportunities that come my way, such as my father, Father Trevor Huddleston, St Margaret's School, Bushey, and "Uncle" Ken. All these influences have helped me to expand my horizons. Incidentally, Father Trevor Huddleston became a Bishop and was elected Archbishop of the Indian Ocean in 1978.

The political interest, which was woken in South Africa, continued through my life as I lived through the Front De Liberation du Quebec (FLQ) crisis in Montreal when I emigrated to Canada in 1970. It blossomed when I moved to Prince George in British Columbia, where I became heavily involved in the Green Party. My involvement continues to this day as I strive to tread lightly on the Earth and work towards equality for all and away from economic growth. The philosophy of Gross National Happiness (GNH) has so much more to offer than the worshipping of Gross National Product (GNP).

MINI SAGA IN SOUTH AFRICA

I continue to attend St Giles Presbyterian Church and take comfort from the teachings and community. I am equally comfortable when I return to the Anglican Church on my visits to England. I am thankful for the religious upbringing I received both from my parents and from St Margaret's School, Bushey. Church was always a very important part of our life. This solid background built a strong foundation and opened my heart and mind to understanding and responding to the greater need.

All these factors combined together to prepare me for recognizing and accepting opportunities that would expand my horizons. I am so thankful for this life and all the wonderful and influential people I have met along the way. We must always endeavour to keep our hearts and minds open to these opportunities and never let fear distract us from the way.

For a long time, my year in South Africa was the best year of my life. As more experiences have accumulated, there have been many more years of wonder and achievement. We can influence our own lives by accepting opportunities and by not letting fear impede any potential life experiences. South Africa continues to be an important and special part of my life.

GLOSSARY:

ANC   African National Congress.

Apartheid   System of separate development by race and colour.

Afrikaans   Language spoken by Afrikaners, who are Dutch descendants. South Africa was bilingual: English and Afrikaans.

Bantu   A linguistic term for a group of African languages, including Zulu, Sotho, Xhosa, Ndebele, and Matabele. In 1960s was term used for Black Africans in South Africa.

Biltong   Jerky.

Bobotie   Malaysian meatloaf.

Boers   White settlers of Dutch descent; Afrikaner agriculturalists.

Boerwoers   Afrikaans sausage.

Black Sash Movement   Group of white women activists opposing Apartheid.

Braivleis   Barbecue.

Community of the Resurrection	Anglican religious order.
Kraal	A grouping of rondavels.
Mealie	Maize when cooked.
Mealie Meal	Corn based porridge or pap.
Rondavel	Round hut with conical thatched roof.
San	Bushmen.
Suffragette	Activist women fighting for women's vote.
uMkhonto we Sizwe	Spear of the Nation. Military wing of ANC.
Veldschoen	Hiking shoes.
Voortrekkers	Afrikaner settlers who trekked inland from the Cape with wagons.

PEOPLE FEATURED IN TEXT:

Alan Paton	South African author.
Archbishop Desmond Tutu	Head of Anglican church in South Africa.
Charles Johnson	Archdeacon of Zululand.
Ken Johnson	Canon of Pietermaritzburg and Zululand.
Daisy Solomon	Suffragette in England. Daughter of the governor of the Cape.
Father Trevor Huddleston	Anglican priest. Member of the Community of the Resurrection.
Harald Pager	Archaeologist of Ndedema Gorge.
Helen Suzman	Leader of Progressive Party of South Africa.
Hugh Prosser	Principal of St Augustine's Mission School in Penhalonga.
Nelson Mandela	Leader of ANC. Prime minister of South Africa.

GEOGRAPHICAL NAME CHANGES:

Grahamstown – Makhanda

Lourenco Marques – Maputo

Natal – KwaZulu Natal

Rhodesia – Zimbabwe

Salisbury – Harare

South West Africa – Namibia

Swaziland – Eswatini

Umtali – Mutare

Umtata – Mthatha

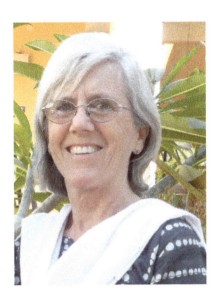

ABOUT THE AUTHOR

Hilary Crowley emigrated to Canada two years after this adventure, where she still lives. She spent many years working as an itinerant physiotherapist in rural communities in British Columbia. She has returned to South Africa several times and has witnessed the changes in the country before and after Apartheid.

In 1994, she spent a year in India helping to develop a community-based rehabilitation program during the height of the polio epidemic. She returned to India annually over a twenty-five-year period to provide further training to the staff and to further develop the program. She founded a charity in Canada to support this program, Samuha Overseas Development Association, S.O.D.A. www.samuha.ca

In 2019, Hilary published her first book about this endeavour, *FOOTSTEPS TO FREEDOM – Tales of Therapy in Rural India.* Hilary also volunteered with medical teams in Tibet, Bhutan, and Ladakh. She published her second book relating these experiences, *HEALTH IN THE HIMALAYA – Tibet Bhutan Ladakh.* Hilary's third travel memoir, *MINI SAGA IN SOUTH AFRICA* narrates her experiences in South Africa, which largely influenced her life path from 1967 to the present day.